## DATE DUE

| | | |
|---|---|---|
| DEC 0 8 2010 | | |
| DEC 1 7 2010 | | |
| JUN 0 7 2012 | | |
| | | |
| | | |
| | | |
| | | |
| | | |
| | | |
| | | |
| | | |
| | | |
| | | |
| | | |
| | | |
| | | |
| | | |
| | | |
| GAYLORD | | PRINTED IN U.S.A. |

# REFORMING MEDICARE

A CENTURY FOUNDATION BOOK

# REFORMING MEDICARE

## Options, Tradeoffs, and Opportunities

HENRY J. AARON

JEANNE M. LAMBREW

*with*

PATRICK F. HEALY

BROOKINGS INSTITUTION PRESS
*Washington, D.C.*

Copyright © 2008
The Century Foundation
All rights reserved. No part of this publication may be reproduced or transmitted in any form or
by any means without permission in writing from the Brookings Institution Press,
1775 Massachusetts Avenue, N.W., Washington, D.C. 20036 (www.brookings.edu; fax
202/536-3623 or e-mail: permissions@brookings.edu)

*Library of Congress Cataloging-in-Publication data*
Aaron, Henry J.
Reforming Medicare : options, tradeoffs, opportunities / Henry J. Aaron and Jeanne M.
Lambrew, Patrick F. Healy.
p.      cm.
"A Century Foundation book."
Includes bibliographical references and index.
Summary: "Identifies and analyzes the three leading approaches to Medicare reform: updated
social insurance, premium support, and consumer-directed Medicare, rating each on its political
viability as well as ability to promote access to health care, improve quality of care, and control
costs. Describes incremental strategies that blend elements of each plan"—Provided by publisher.
ISBN 978-0-8157-0124-8 (cloth : alk. paper)
1. Medicare. 2. Health care reform—United States. 3. Medical policy—United States.
I. Lambrew, Jeanne M. II. Healey, Patrick F. (Patrick Ferrigan), 1982– III. Century Foundation.
IV. Brookings Institution. V. Title.
[DNLM: 1. Medicare—organization & administration. 2. Health Care Reform—organization
& administration—United States. 3. Health Policy—United States. WT 31 A111r 2008]
RA412.3.A27 2008
368.4'2600973—dc22                                                                2008018709

9 8 7 6 5 4 3 2 1

The paper used in this publication meets minimum requirements of the
American National Standard for Information Sciences—Permanence of Paper for
Printed Library Materials: ANSI Z39.48-1992.

Typeset in Adobe Garamond

Composition by Peter Lindeman
Arlington, Virginia

Printed by R. R. Donnelley
Harrisonburg, Virginia

# Contents

# Foreword

Some day, looking back, this period will be recalled as part of a great transformation in American life. The watershed represented by the aging of 76 million baby boomers will alter tastes in entertainment, transform our politics, and reshape the economy. Older people, after all, have quite different consumption preferences than the young. To be flip about it: they buy walkers instead of skateboards and dentures rather than braces. They also buy lots of health services—more all the time.

The American way of providing health care is expensive, but it is innovative. It is unequal, but at the top it provides some of the best care in the world. Despite the sharp cost increases in the recent past and the dire projections of continued growth in health care expenditures, the pressure to make more services available is intense, particularly among older Americans. The impetus provided by an aging population and the steady development of new products seems unstoppable. But the simple arithmetic of the trends suggests that something important is going to have to change—whether most people like it or not.

The past several years have seen debates intensify concerning many areas of health care—scientific issues in medical practice, prescription drugs, emergency room use, and end-of-life care, to name a few—and underlying most of these conflicts is the unusual way we pay for health care in the United States. Statistically, our approach involves spending much more than other industrialized countries do for results that are often no better and in many cases worse. Americans actually have been relatively passive about the considerable evidence that we are getting mediocre health care outcomes compared to other countries. In fact, there is intense opposition to adapting the American system so that it reflects more of the efficiencies of modern European approaches.

In the dozen years since President Clinton's proposal for universal health insurance failed to become law, Congress has focused mainly on reforming the Medicare and Medicaid programs that provide coverage to older and low-income Americans. The most notable achievement during that time, the addition of Medicare Part D, covering prescription drugs, was an especially important expansion of benefits.

One basic point about the Medicare debate is quite straightforward: although there are those who would like to scrap the program completely and shift to a market-based system, people who actually run for office overwhelmingly talk about strengthening and saving, not replacing, the program. Medicare, in other words, has strong political backing among the millions of Americans who depend on it for health care.

In this volume, two of the nation's leading experts on the social safety net—Henry J. Aaron, senior fellow in economic studies and the Bruce and Virginia MacLaury Chair at the Brookings Institution, and Jeanne M. Lambrew, associate professor of public affairs at the Lyndon B. Johnson School of Public Affairs, University of Texas–Austin, and a senior fellow at the Center for American Progress—provide a comprehensive look at Medicare today, its prospects for tomorrow, and the options for dealing with the challenges to the program. The authors provide a balanced analysis of the pros and cons of each general approach for reforming the program. In so doing, they put forward a framework for serious debate about which approach (or mix of approaches) would serve Americans best.

Ultimately, as the authors acknowledge, the conclusions that readers reach about the best strategy for reforming Medicare will more likely derive from their personal values and beliefs than from the research and analysis presented in this volume. Indeed, one of the great benefits of Aaron and Lambrew's book is that it provides the most useful available information buttressing the case for each side of the debate.

The Century Foundation has published a number of works in this area in recent years. Most recently, we released Arnold S. Relman's *A Second*

*Opinion: Rescuing America's Health Care.* Our previous projects include David J. Rothman's *Beginnings Count: The Technological Imperative in American Health Care;* Charles R. Morris's *Too Much of a Good Thing? Why Health Care Spending Won't Make Us Sick* and *Apart at the Seams: The Collapse of Private Pension and Health Care Protections; Medicare Tomorrow: The Report of The Century Foundation Task Force on Medicare Reform;* and Leif Wellington Haase's *A New Deal for Health: How to Cover Everyone and Get Medical Costs under Control.*

We are especially pleased that this comprehensive volume is appearing in the midst of a presidential campaign, when political rhetoric about an issue as complex as Medicare—and health care generally—can leave voters confused about which side's case is most persuasive. Regardless of who wins in November, Medicare reform will almost certainly be high on the agenda of the new administration and Congress. Let us hope that the clarity and objectivity that characterize this book will be reflected in the debates and outcome in Washington.

On behalf of the Trustees of the Century Foundation, I thank Henry Aaron and Jeanne Lambrew for their efforts. They, in turn, wish to thank Robert Reischauer who read and reviewed much of the book, Melissa Cox, who helped during the initial stages of research, Vicky Macintyre for editing the manuscript, Kathleen Elliott Yinug for administrative support, and three anonymous referees for constructive and extensive criticisms and suggestions.

RICHARD C. LEONE, *President*
The Century Foundation

# 1 | Medicare Reform: The Stakes

Now in its fifth decade, Medicare provides health coverage to virtually all of the nation's elderly and a large share of people with disabilities, a population of some 44 million. The program has brought large benefits.[1] With dramatically improved access to health care, its beneficiaries have enjoyed longer, healthier lives.[2] It contributed to the desegregation of southern hospitals. And it is one of the most popular government programs, rivaling Social Security.

Despite Medicare's achievements and popularity, the program has always been controversial. In the bitter partisan dispute preceding its enactment, Democrats supported mandatory, payroll-tax-financed hospital care while Republicans sought voluntary, premium-, and tax-financed coverage of doctors' services. Physicians opposed both ideas, fearing government intrusion into medical practice. To appease them, the final plan required the government to pay all reasonable hospital costs and customary physician fees. That policy mollified providers but fueled rapid increases in hospital spending and doctors' fees. Soon, program outlays far outpaced original projections, and

Medicare was blamed for causing health care inflation. So, starting in the early 1980s, Congress required Medicare to pay health care providers in new ways designed to hold down spending. In the 1990s Congress enacted additional major payment cutbacks, but angry protests from aggrieved hospital and private plan administrators, among others, forced it to reverse many of these cuts. More recent concerns have focused on physician fees, rising expenditures, and overpayments to managed care plans.

Some of the debate also focuses on benefit limits imposed to hold down projected costs. To circumvent these limits, most Medicare enrollees have bought supplemental insurance to cover deductibles, cost sharing, and such excluded services as outpatient prescription drugs and long-term care. In 1988 Congress moved to fill the prescription drug gap. However, the law was so unpopular with beneficiaries that Congress repealed it little more than a year after enactment. Not until 2003 did Congress succeed in adding this service, long a feature of private health insurance plans. That bill also aroused intense controversy because of its design, administration, and manner of passage. It will be a source of debate for years to come.

Another looming issue is whether and how to change Medicare to deal with population aging and the proliferation of beneficial but costly interventions. These trends guarantee that Medicare spending will far outpace the growth of federal revenues and thereby increase the burden for those who pay for most of the program's costs—namely, taxpayers. Beneficiaries will face mounting challenges too, for they shoulder roughly one-fifth of the cost of the care they use. To complicate matters, the quality of services provided to all Americans, including Medicare beneficiaries, is deficient in important respects: as is well documented, errors are too common, and recommended care is frequently not rendered.[3]

Rising costs, limited access, and deficient quality are not the only problems. Considerable confusion arises in debates about health care policy in general, and Medicare in particular, because they combine issues from economics, politics, psychology, and medical science. Moreover, the stakes for all parties—patients, providers, insurers, and taxpayers—are high. The outcome will affect millions of people and involve trillions of dollars. To aid in understanding Medicare's complexities and assessing major policy proposals, this book offers a program "primer," describing its history, principal goals, operation, and future challenges.

## Born in Turmoil

Medicare and Medicaid became law on the afternoon of July 31, 1965, at a signing ceremony in Independence, Missouri. President Lyndon B. Johnson had decided a few days before to move the event from Washington to Independence, the site of the library of former president Harry S. Truman. Johnson wanted to honor Truman for trying to win passage of national health insurance. Although that effort was entirely without success, it started the lengthy political process that led to congressional approval of Medicare and Medicaid. Explaining the move to Wilbur Cohen, the administration's point man for crafting the legislation, Johnson said: "Don't you understand? I'm doing this for Harry Truman. He's old and he's tired and he's been left all alone down there. I want him to know that his country has not forgotten him. I wonder if anyone will do the same for me."[4]

The signing took place before thirty-three members of Congress and numerous other officials and citizens. Johnson sat at the same small table President Truman had used in 1947 when he signed the Truman Doctrine legislation that initiated aid to Greece and Turkey. The former president gave a brief welcoming speech, declaring his pleasure at having lived to see the signing of the bill. Johnson expressed pride that the bill had passed during his administration and thanked the invited guests who had contributed to its passage. He used 72 pens to sign his name. He gave the first pen to Truman, the second to Truman's wife, and the remainder, plus an additional 150 pens, to other guests. The entire ceremony lasted only twenty minutes.[5] Brief and bland, it belied the rancorous and protracted political maneuvering that preceded it.

The first serious bill to promise universal health insurance was introduced in 1939, during Franklin Roosevelt's second term. With metronomic regularity, similar bills were reintroduced in each succeeding Congress and ignored. No hearings were even held on the proposal President Truman endorsed in 1949.

When John Kennedy tried to deliver on a campaign promise of hospital insurance for the elderly, the idea failed to win approval in the House Committee on Ways and Means. The committee's formidable chairman, Wilbur Mills (D-Ark.), knew that he lacked the votes to move the bill (it was not even clear that he wanted to do so). The majority of the committee, which comprised conservative Republicans and southern Democrats, strongly opposed the Democratic proposal for hospital insurance financed by a mandatory payroll tax. The Republicans favored a voluntary, premium-, and tax-financed plan to cover physician bills. The southern Democrats feared—correctly, as events later proved—that federal payment for hospital services would help enforce equal access for blacks and whites in the still-segregated South.

Then came President Kennedy's assassination and the Democratic landslide of 1964. Many members of the enlarged Democratic majority hailed from northern and western states. They were disposed to support Medicare on the House floor. Some took seats on the Ways and Means Committee. It became clear that hospital insurance might pass the Ways and Means Committee even without Mills's support. Instead of opposing the bill, however, Mills designed a compromise that combined mandatory hospital insurance financed by payroll taxes (the Democrats' plan) with voluntary coverage of physicians' services financed by premiums and general revenues and extended means-tested health coverage of the poor (the Republicans' plan). The first two components constitute Medicare, the third Medicaid.

The original hospital insurance proposal met with strident criticism from other quarters as well. Some said Medicare would deny patients the freedom to seek the kind of care they wanted and would stop physicians from practicing medicine as they thought best. The president of the American Medical Association (AMA), Donovan Ward, likened the AMA's fight against Medicare to Winston Churchill's stand against the Nazis.[6] He labeled the plan a deception that would endanger the relationship between patients and doctors. According to Milford O. Rouse, speaker of the House of Delegates of the AMA, the battle to defeat Medicare was a battle for "the American way of life" and "the protection of the sick."[7] Perhaps the most eloquent attack came from a politically active movie actor named Ronald Reagan, who warned that Medicare would invite socialism to "invade every area of freedom in this country" and force Americans to spend their "sunset years telling our children and our children's children what it was like in America when men were free."[8] These jarring attacks embodied a political ideology that continues to fuel some criticisms of Medicare.[9]

The House approved the bill 313-115. A somewhat different version passed the Senate 68-21. The House-Senate conference compromise was passed with similar majorities.[10] Actuarial estimates put the cost of the final plan at $3 billion a year (about $19 billion in 2007 dollars).[11]

## History after Enactment

Since 1965, the character of health insurance in the United States has changed greatly. Health maintenance organizations and managed care have recast the typical job-based health plan. Private plans have linked insurance and delivery of care. In contrast, Medicare's system of parallel but separate plans—called Hospital Insurance (HI, or Part A) and Supplementary Medical Insurance (SMI, or Part B)—preserve the typical 1965 insurance configuration of the separate Blue Cross and Blue Shield plans. The major changes have been the addition of managed care (Part C), as an alternative to Parts A and B, and an outpatient prescription drug benefit (Part D).

Whereas private insurance has become more integrated, Medicare has been slow to adapt to changing medical practice, beneficiary needs, and societal expectations. Decades passed before the program covered outpatient prescription drugs and preventive services that are of increasing importance to the elderly and people with disabilities. It still provides minimal coverage of mental health care and nursing home stays that do not follow hospitalization. And it does not cap out-of-pocket spending, now a benefit under most employer-sponsored plans. To fill these gaps, as well as to reduce Medicare's steep cost sharing, most beneficiaries seek supplemental protection. Some supplemental coverage comes from former employers or unions and some from individual purchase of so-called Medigap insurance. Many poor Medicare beneficiaries are also dually eligible for Medicaid, which pays for premiums, cost sharing, and additional services.

Although the growth of per capita Medicare spending has paralleled that of private insurance, Medicare spending has outpaced other federal spending. Moreover, Part A spending has grown faster than dedicated revenues, causing periodic "trust fund crises." These trust fund imbalances as well as Medicare's benefit gaps have triggered three major changes and small modifications since 1965.

### *Catastrophic Coverage Act of 1988*

In 1988 Congress enacted the Medicare Catastrophic Coverage Act (P.L. 100-360). The title referred to the bill's coverage of large outlays but ironically turned out to describe the law's political fate. Proposed by the Reagan administration, the new law was passed by a Democratic Congress with bipartisan support. Among its numerous benefits, the act lowered deductibles and removed coinsurance and time limits on hospital coverage, increased skilled nursing home coverage, removed all limits on hospice coverage, and covered outpatient prescription drugs above a deductible. The full cost of these added benefits was offset by an added premium paid by roughly 40 percent of Medicare enrollees with the highest personal incomes.

Having yielded to the pressures of both the Republican administration (which wanted beneficiaries to pay all of the added cost of the new benefits) and the Democratic Congress (which wanted progressive financing), the financing scheme doomed the entire law. Most of the cost of the new benefits fell on a minority of Medicare beneficiaries, many of whom were slated to pay far more in taxes than the value of the benefits they received. Others mistakenly thought that they were net losers. Many Medicare enrollees already had most of the new benefits from former employers. For them, the bill brought nothing but higher premiums. Worse still, premium increases were to take effect before the new benefits were available. The putative beneficiaries protested loudly and, on occasion, violently. Just sixteen months after its enactment, Congress overwhelmingly repealed the law.[12]

### The Balanced Budget Act of 1997

The next several years saw a pair of major proposals and setbacks for both parties. President Bill Clinton proposed to cut Medicare's payment rates and add a drug benefit in his 1993 health reform plan. These Medicare changes died along with the rest of the plan in 1994. In 1995 the newly ascendant Republican congressional majority tried to cap Medicare outlays and lower spending by an estimated $270 billion over seven years. Clinton vetoed the bill containing this provision, but he put forward a compromise proposal that led to bipartisan legislation in 1997.[13]

Official projections that year indicated the HI trust fund would be insolvent in 2001.[14] To forestall that event and reduce the overall federal budget deficit, Congress enacted the Balanced Budget Act of 1997 (P.L. 105-33). Unlike virtually any Medicare legislation before or since, it was hailed as a victory by both parties. This bill included reductions in the growth of provider payments. It shifted some Hospital Insurance (Part A) costs to Supplementary Medical Insurance (Part B), lessening pressure on the payroll-tax-financed HI trust fund but forcing Part B premium increases. The bill also intensified official efforts to root out inappropriate and fraudulent payments to providers. It improved preventive benefits and low-income beneficiary protections and created a Medicare commission to identify policy ideas for the program's long-term challenges.

Following this legislation, nominal Medicare expenditures per beneficiary fell in 1998, the first absolute decline since the program was enacted. Responding to provider complaints, Congress repeatedly raised reimbursement rates.[15] Even with these "give-backs," the bill pushed back by twenty-eight years the date of insolvency for the Hospital Insurance program according to the 2001 Annual Report of the Medicare Trustees.[16]

### The Medicare Modernization Act of 2003

Aside from the Catastrophic Coverage Act, most Medicare legislation before 2003 was triggered by projected insolvency in the HI trust fund or by overall budget deficits. Typically, such legislation modestly altered the program and left no lasting political rancor. In contrast, the Medicare Modernization Act of 2003 (MMA, P.L. 108-173) significantly changed Medicare, and its manner of passage aroused resentments that will shadow future Medicare reform efforts.

Focusing on his 2004 reelection challenge, President George W. Bush made passage of a prescription drug benefit a top legislative priority for 2003. By leading a successful effort to improve Medicare, the president hoped to show that a Republican-controlled executive and legislature could deliver on a promise made often, but never fulfilled, to extend Medicare to cover prescription drugs. He also pledged to advance a conservative vision by linking high-deductible plans to health savings accounts and by encouraging enrollment in private Medicare plans.

In June 2003 the House and Senate passed different versions of the legislation. The House, divided along party lines, produced a bill closely resembling President Bush's vision. The Senate bill drew bipartisan support. Under normal procedure, a conference committee including both Republicans and Democrats from both chambers would have fashioned a compromise that both houses could pass. In this case, however, the Republican majority invited no House Democrats to participate and only two Senate Democrats—Max Baucus (Mont.) and John Breaux (La.)—both of whom accepted aspects of the House bill that most Senate Democrats opposed. Financial considerations further complicated negotiations: the total cost of the bill could not exceed $400 billion, a ten-year spending limit imposed by the budget resolution of fiscal 2004.[17] Despite these snags, the conference committee completed its work in November 2003.

However, passage was not assured. Most Democrats remained strongly opposed to the bill. Some Republicans also rejected any increase in a program they regarded as already careening toward insolvency; others thought that the final compromise emasculated provisions in the House bill designed to promote competition. House floor debate was acrimonious, initially presaging defeat. But the Republican leadership extended the usual fifteen-minute voting period to almost three hours, during which it rounded up a narrow, largely partisan, majority.[18] House Democrats were furious but helpless. Senate debate was no less contentious, because Democrats believed that they had been inadequately represented in conference. In the end, however, enough Democrats joined the Republican majority to pass the bill, expanding Medicare's benefit package to include outpatient prescription drugs.[19]

The benefit (see chapter 2) is delivered in two ways: through stand-alone prescription drug plans (christened Part D) or through Medicare Advantage plans (Part C). The MMA also increased payments to private plans to promote them as an alternative to the traditional fee-for-service delivery system. In addition, the MMA changed provider payment rates, took some small steps toward rewarding quality care, and began to explore the potential of disease management. It also established a new measure of program insolvency based on the proportion of total outlays covered by general revenues.[20]

The passage of the MMA did little to quell controversy. Representative Nick Smith (R-Mich.) charged that he had been threatened and offered a bribe during the three-hour-long vote.[21] In March 2004 Medicare's chief actuary complained that during the negotiations leading to the final compromise he had been forbidden by Tom Scully, administrator of the Centers for Medicare and Medicaid Services (CMS) and a political appointee, to share with Congress his estimate that the bill would cost $534 billion for the period 2004–13.[22] Had the actuary's estimate—which was much more than the $400 billion authorized in the fiscal 2004 budget resolution and the $395 billion estimate of the Congressional Budget Office (CBO)—been made public, the conference agreement would likely have been defeated. After the bill was enacted, Democrats charged that the television ads, fliers, and news videos the administration prepared to inform seniors of their new options were misleading and represented veiled political propaganda. When the Government Accountability Office concluded that some of the videos were an illegal "covert form of propaganda," the administration stopped their use.[23]

Once the drug benefit went into effect in 2006, its implementation was relatively smooth. Within a year, all areas of the country had a private drug plan, enrollment rose, beneficiary satisfaction was high, and expenditures turned out to be lower than originally projected by both the CBO and

CMS. Even so, the MMA continues to be hotly debated, particularly because of its prohibition on government involvement in drug price negotiation and the role of private plans in Medicare. In all likelihood, its new insolvency measure will provoke new debates on how to reform the system.

## Future Challenges

Medicare has by and large met its goals of providing affordable access to health care for the elderly and persons with disabilities (see chapter 3). Moreover, access is comparable to that provided by private insurance, and the growth in per capita spending is close to that of private plans. As for satisfaction, a 2001 survey found elderly Medicare beneficiaries nearly three times more likely than enrollees in employer-sponsored plans to rate their health insurance as excellent.[24]

All the same, Medicare policy will no doubt invite further debate. Many continue to object to government-managed health insurance on principle. Others still question whether Medicare covers too much or too little of its beneficiaries' health expenditures. And a good number balk at growing program outlays.[25] Cost-containment efforts, precipitated in the past by the desire to limit federal spending and by projected insolvency of the HI trust fund, will now focus on the degree to which the entire program relies on general revenues.

### Cost

Between 2008 and 2018, Medicare's share of non-interest federal spending is expected to rise from 14.8 to 17.1 percent.[26] As a result, the program will put steadily increasing pressure on the rest of the government budget (chapter 3). The MMA intensified those pressures, widening the projected federal budget deficit by an average of 1 percent of gross domestic product over the succeeding seventy-five years.[27]

Fast-rising costs are bound to impose major new burdens on individual beneficiaries, as well as taxpayers. Out-of-pocket spending on health care for seniors equals about 45 percent of their Social Security benefits and could surpass 60 percent by 2030.[28] These shares will be even higher for those with above-average medical expenditures. If rising outlays buy services that are worth what they cost, they will signal a huge increase in the well-being of Medicare beneficiaries due to improved health care services. Even so, the financial readjustments necessary to divert resources to Medicare will be troublesome.

*Access*

The modest expansion of Medicare's covered services has failed to allay concerns about benefit adequacy. Cost sharing for some services remains high. The duration of coverage for hospital and skilled nursing home stays is limited. Before enactment of the MMA, Medicare covered nearly half of the health and long-term care expenses of its beneficiaries.[29] As detailed in chapter 2, beneficiaries have to pay premiums, deductibles, and other cost sharing, not to mention fees for uncovered services. Those with serious medical problems can incur catastrophic out-of-pocket expenses if they do not have supplemental coverage.

Such insurance has become increasingly costly and hard to find. These trends are likely to continue. A 1990 decision of the Financial Accounting Standards Board required businesses to recognize on their balance sheets a liability for the present value of projected medical benefits for their current and future retirees.[30] A similar policy is going into effect for the public sector, which has historically provided retiree coverage. Although the liabilities are not new, their heightened prominence on private employers' balance sheets is thought to depress share values. Accordingly, many businesses have curtailed or discontinued once-generous retiree health benefits. The proportion of large firms offering retiree health coverage fell from 66 percent in 1988 to 33 percent in 2007.[31] Many retirees who still have employer-sponsored policies are seeing a sharp increase in premiums and co-payments—10 percent in 2006, even with the addition of the drug benefit.[32] Medigap, too, has been on the decline, as fewer seniors have been able to afford its premiums.

## Plan of the Book

For those who are not familiar with the Medicare program, we begin in chapter 2 with a detailed description of Medicare's structure and financing. Readers who are generally familiar with how Medicare works are advised to skip chapter 2. Chapter 3 assesses the program's current performance in providing affordable, accessible, high-quality coverage. Next, we take up three strategies for program reform (chapters 4–6): updated social insurance, which would retain the current system while rationalizing coverage and reducing bureaucracy; premium support to replace the current system with a capped, per person payment that beneficiaries could use to buy health insurance; and consumer-directed Medicare, wherein beneficiaries would pay for care up to a high deductible from government-supported savings accounts and receive premium-support coverage above the deductible. We then evaluate these strategies against program objectives and rate their political strengths and weaknesses (chapter 7).

# 2 A Medicare Primer

Since its enactment in 1965, Medicare has expanded from two to four components. The first offerings were Hospital Insurance (HI, or Part A) and Supplementary Medical Insurance covering physicians and other selected services (SMI, or Part B).[1] In 1982 Congress added coverage of managed care plans (now named Medicare Advantage, or Part C). In 2003 it approved coverage of outpatient prescription drugs through privately administered insurance plans (Part D).

The basic structure of Parts A and B has not changed since enactment. It remains a fee-for-service system that allows enrollees to select virtually any licensed provider and receive any covered service they and their providers deem appropriate. In contrast, most private insurance plans have adopted administrative practices to hold down costs, including care management, utilization reviews, and selective provider networks to leverage lower prices.

The program has changed in several other important respects, however. In 1972 eligibility for Medicare benefits was extended to those receiving Social Security Disability Insurance pensions (after a two-year waiting period) and to victims of end-stage renal disease.[2] In a pioneering move, it introduced prospective payment of most hospitals, physicians, and other providers in place of reimbursements based largely on costs or customary charges. In addition, it offered new benefits, including hospice care (first covered in 1983) and various preventive services, such as screening for colon and breast cancer and flu shots.

## Who Is Covered

In 2007 Medicare covered an average 44.1 million people a month—36.9 million elderly, 7.2 million people with disabilities, and approximately 223,000 with renal failure.[3] Expenditures for that year totaled $432 billion.[4]

Before Medicare, only about half of the elderly had health insurance. Coverage was often narrow.[5] People whose health had deteriorated could have their coverage canceled or premiums increased. Initially, Medicare covered everyone aged sixty-five or older. Part A now covers anyone aged sixty-five or older who has worked for ten years or more in employment subject to the Medicare payroll tax.[6] It also covers their spouses or former spouses at age sixty-five. Most of the Medicare population is female, white, between the ages of sixty-five and eighty-four, in good or fair health, and living with a spouse.

Part A eligibles may also enroll in Part B, which covers primarily outpatient and physician care. Anyone enrolled in Part A or Part B may buy subsidized prescription drug coverage under Part D.[7] Most Part B enrollees must pay a premium that covers just one-fourth of Part B costs. The basic premium was $96.40 a month in 2008.[8] The 75 percent subsidy helps explain why 94 percent of those eligible to buy Part B coverage do so.[9] Beginning in 2007, upper-income beneficiaries were required to pay premiums covering more than one-fourth of the cost of their insurance: the income threshold was $80,000 for single Part B participants and $160,000 for couples.[10] At that point, only about 4 percent of Part B enrollees faced increased premiums.[11] The increased premiums had little impact on participation in Part B, at least initially, because few people were affected and because Medicare enjoys other marketing advantages.[12] Participation may decline, however, if either the number of seniors facing extra premiums grows rapidly or the premium itself begins to constitute a sizable share of their income.

Roughly one Medicare beneficiary in five elects to enroll in a Medicare Advantage (MA) plan rather than receive care through the traditional fee-for-service delivery system.[13] To be eligible for an MA plan, a beneficiary must be enrolled in Medicare Parts A and B, must live in the service area of the MA plan, and cannot have end-stage renal disease at the time of

Table 2-1. *Medicare Spending per Beneficiary, 2004*

| Category | Dollar amount |
|---|---|
| All beneficiaries | 7,121 |
| Dual-eligible[a] | 10,884 |
| Non-dual-eligible | 5,975 |
| Disabled (non-end-stage renal disease) | 6,023 |
| Elderly | 6,782 |
|   65–74 | 5,226 |
|   75–84 | 8,059 |
|   ≥ 85 | 10,765 |
| End-stage renal disease | 54,370 |
| Excellent health | 4,082 |
| Good or fair health | 7,943 |
| Poor health | 15,448 |

Source: MedPAC analysis of the Medicare Current Beneficiary Survey, Cost and Use file, 2004. MedPAC, *A Data Book: Healthcare Spending and the Medicare Program* (June 2007).
a. Persons who are entitled to Medicare (Part A or Part B) and who are also eligible for Medicaid.

enrollment.[14] Medicare pays these plans fixed monthly amounts per enrollee that vary according to the participant's age, sex, health characteristics, and county of residence. Historically, enrollees in Medicare Advantage were healthier and younger than those who remained in traditional Medicare, although the differences are narrowing as more beneficiaries enroll in private plans.

Not surprisingly, Medicare spends the most on the sick, old, and poor (see table 2-1). Overall, Medicare spending accounted for 45 percent of total spending on medical and long-term care services by its beneficiaries in 2002. Private insurance—primarily employer-sponsored retiree coverage and individually purchased Medigap plans—paid 18 percent of beneficiaries' costs. Medicaid and other public sources of coverage paid 12 and 6 percent of beneficiaries' costs, respectively. Beneficiaries paid 19 percent of their health and long-term care costs out of pocket.[15]

## What Is Covered

Congress defines the categories of services that Medicare covers, but administrative officials determine what the categories include. Congress is reluctant to add more categories because congressional rules require that legislation increasing program outlays identify ways to pay for these extensions and thus must compete against other demands on limited resources. Administrative extensions are not subject to these rules. Spending has risen rapidly in large part because scientific advances have continuously enlarged the content of service categories. As a result, authorities have tried to limit Medicare expenditures by controlling service prices, its primary tool. These efforts have generated rules of mind-bending complexity and created tension between the program and providers.

Initially, Medicare paid hospitals and physicians on the basis of actual charges or costs, a system that fueled rapid price increases. In the 1980s Medicare began to replace that system with prospectively set, fixed payments based on what efficient providers could be *expected* to do rather than on what they *actually* did. Prospective payment was implemented first for inpatient hospital services (1983), then for physicians (1992), skilled nursing facilities (SNFs, 1998), outpatient hospital services and home health agencies (2000), and rehabilitation facilities and long-term care hospitals (2002). The growing concern that the United States does not get as much as it should for its health care spending has led to experiments to determine whether tying payments to outcomes can change what doctors do. These experiments remain incomplete and inconclusive and have not had much effect on the program. The following sections describe each of Medicare's major service categories—what is covered, how payment systems work, the extent of quality monitoring, costs, and supplemental coverage options.

## Inpatient Hospital Care

Each year, roughly one-fifth of Medicare beneficiaries are admitted to an acute-care hospital.[16] Beneficiaries must pay an annual deductible set at the national average daily charge for hospital room and board—$1,024 for 2008. This amount is higher than the deductibles of most private insurance plans. Medicare then covers all costs of the first sixty days of each hospital stay and three-quarters of the cost of the next thirty days. For the small proportion of patients whose hospital stay lasts more than ninety days in a year, Medicare provides an additional nonrenewable lifetime reserve of sixty days of coverage during which patients must pay half the daily charge. Deductible and co-payment liabilities for inpatient hospital services at this point would be formidable for those without significant savings or supplemental insurance—$39,424 in 2008.[17] Medicare provides no further hospital coverage.

PROSPECTIVE PAYMENTS. Medicare typically makes a bundled payment for certain conditions and treatments of inpatients, called diagnosis-related groups (DRGs)—congestive heart failure or a day's care in a nursing home, for example. In 2008 Medicare recognized 744 severity-adjusted DRGs.[18] Medicare also pays for care in three special kinds of hospitals: long-term care hospitals, inpatient rehabilitation facilities, and inpatient psychiatric facilities (see appendix A). The per discharge payments are based on patients' sex, age, diagnoses, co-morbidities and complications, discharge destination, the procedures administered, and local hospital costs, which vary widely.[19] This form of payment is intended to encourage institutional providers to limit lengths of stay and economize on the number and costs of services.

ADDITIONAL PAYMENTS. Hospitals receive outlier payments for extraordinarily costly patients.[20] Teaching hospitals receive extra payments to defray the direct and indirect costs of graduate medical education.[21] Another payment covers the estimated costs of uncompensated hospital care.[22] Many rural hospitals receive extra payments.[23] For example, so-called critical-access hospitals may be paid on the basis of cost rather than DRGs.[24] The purpose of these payments is to support the continued operation of facilities that would otherwise find it hard to remain in operation in thinly settled areas. Finally, hospitals receive add-on payments for cases using certain approved new technologies whose costs are not yet reflected in the base DRG payments.

### Outpatient Hospital Services and Ambulatory Surgery

Part B of Medicare pays some of the cost of services rendered through hospital outpatient departments, including emergency room care, surgery, and laboratory tests. It also covers outpatient physical therapy and rehabilitation, durable medical equipment, chemotherapy, and radiation.[25] Medicare implemented a prospective payment system for outpatient services in August 2000.[26] The system sets payments for individual services using a set of relative weights, an annually updated conversion factor, and adjustments for geographic differences in input prices. Hospitals can also receive outlier payments for unusually costly services and pass-through payments for new technologies. The complexity of this system illustrates the inescapable problems of a payment system that requires separate prices for the myriad activities that characterize modern medical care (see appendix B).

### Hospice Care

Since 1983, Medicare has covered hospice care. Hospices provide palliative care such as nursing, drugs, home health aides, counseling, physician services, short hospital stays, respite care to relieve relatives of care burdens, and other services.[27] Patients whose life expectancy is six months or less as certified by a physician are eligible. Except for nominal drug co-payments, patients bear no costs for hospice care.

One-third of Medicare decedents in 2004 used hospice services.[28] It was long assumed that the hospice program reduced Medicare spending by curbing the use of expensive heroic interventions in the last year of life. Recent analysis contradicts that assumption. On average, expenditures on hospice participants are 4 percent greater than on those who use only traditional medical care, the costs increasing with age and for diseases other than cancer.[29]

### Skilled Nursing Facilities

Medicare covers postacute care for beneficiaries who have spent at least three days in a hospital. They are eligible for assistance with up to 100 days of follow-up care in a skilled nursing facility.[30] Medicare pays fully for the first 20 days and about three-fifths of the cost for the next 80 days of care.[31] Patients bear the full cost of longer SNF stays.[32] Since 1998, Medicare has paid SNFs flat fees adjusted for geographic differences in labor costs and case mix using a system based on resource utilization groups. This system replaced a cost-based system that had led to the proliferation of service use.[33]

### Home Health Services

Medicare covers home health services more generously than the average employer-sponsored health insurance plan does.[34] Coverage is unlimited if it is medically necessary and provided under a plan of care directed by a physician.[35] Beneficiaries face no deductibles or co-payments for these services. Not surprisingly, eligibility for home health benefits has been subject to extensive litigation and administrative changes that have profoundly influenced the number of beneficiaries served, as well as the costs.[36] Between 1989, when a court decision relaxed eligibility criteria, and 1997, when legislation and administrative measures began to restrict access, the number of participants receiving home health services more than doubled, the number of visits per user more than tripled, and outlays rose more than sevenfold.[37] The Balanced Budget Act of 1997 (BBA) imposed new eligibility restrictions on home health, introduced an interim payment system based upon costs with limits, and mandated a prospective payment system, which began operation in October 2000.[38] The BBA had a dramatic effect on the industry; by 2000 the number of beneficiaries served fell by one-third, the number of visits per user fell by half, outlays by half, and the number of agencies by one-third.[39] After implementation of the prospective payment system, however, some of these trends reversed. Between 2000 and 2006, the number of users rose nearly one-fifth, outlays rose by half, and the number of agencies by one-third. And although the number of visits per user fell by about 8 percent over this period, the skill mix of services shifted to a much higher level than that furnished before 2000.[40]

### Physician and Other Health Professional Services

The payment of physicians has tightened considerably since Medicare's creation. Initially, payment rules were lax because legislators feared doctors and other providers might boycott the program, especially in view of the fierce opposition to its enactment by the American Medical Association and others in the medical community. Whether on not these fears were overblown, the lax rules ensured the participation of virtually all physicians and other health professionals. Medicare payments now account for more than 20 percent of all physicians' revenues.[41] Although the payment system has been tightened, 80 percent of physicians accepted all or most new Medicare patients in 2006, and only 3 percent accepted none.[42]

Part B of Medicare covers physician visits without limit. Patients must meet an annual deductible—$135 in 2008.[43] Thereafter, Medicare pays 80 percent of an established fee schedule for medical services and 50 percent for mental health services.[44] Physicians who accept the Medicare payment and forgo billing patients are called "participating" physicians; they are paid faster and receive a 5 percent bonus payment.[45] Patients are responsible for charges by nonparticipating physicians above the schedule amount, up to a limit.[46]

FEES. From 1966 to 1991, Medicare paid any physician fees characterized as "usual, customary, and reasonable."[47] This system contributed to growth of per beneficiary spending on physician services under Part B, which averaged 10 percent a year in that period. In 1992, Medicare shifted to the resource-based-relative-value-scale (RBRVS) system. It relates fees to the amount of work required to provide a service, expenses related to maintaining a practice, liability insurance costs, and the geographic location of the provider (see box 2-1).

OVERALL LIMITS: SUSTAINABLE GROWTH RATE SYSTEM. The RBRVS system anchors physician fees to estimated practice costs but does not limit the number of visits or intensity of service. To hold down physician payments, Congress in 1997 adopted the sustainable growth rate (SGR) sys-

Box 2-1. *How RBRVS Works*

RBRVS fees are based on three factors: (1) "relative value units" (RVUs) that measure the relative cost of providing different services, (2) geographic adjustments that reflect differences across market areas in the cost of producing care, and (3) a conversion factor, which ensures that overall spending meets predetermined national targets.

With the help of panels of physicians, Medicare estimates three RVUs for each of nearly 7,000 services.[1] One measures the levels of time, effort, skill, and stress a physician must devote to providing the particular service in comparison with the average service. A second measures relative practice expenses associated with the office, such as rent, supplies, and administrative salaries. The third measures malpractice insurance costs. Each RVU is multiplied by an adjustment factor that measures geographic differences in the costs of labor, non-labor office expenses, or malpractice insurance. Each year, these multipliers are computed for the ninety-nine geographical areas. The sum of the products of the RVUs and geographic adjustment factors is then multiplied by a flat dollar amount, the "conversion factor," which was $37.8975 in 2007.

1. CMS, "Estimated Sustainable Growth Rate and Conversion Factor, for Medicare Payments to Physicians in 2009" (www.cms.hhs.gov/SustainableGRatesConFact).

tem. Because this convoluted system is a continuing source of debate, we provide a detailed explanation of its operation in appendix C. It is important to note here that the SGR formula has implied sizable reductions in physician fees in recent years. According to Medicare actuary estimates, physician payments per service under the SGR will decrease by 5 percent a year through at least 2016.[48]

QUALITY. Under the Tax Relief and Health Care Act of 2006, Congress approved a system of reporting physician quality, to be managed by Medicare.[49] Although the legislation allowed physicians to report quality data on a voluntary basis, it tied payment increases to the reporting system. Thus participating eligible professionals who report data may earn a bonus.[50]

*Other Services*

Medicare pays for clinical laboratory services with no cost sharing by beneficiaries (for details on payment methodology, see appendix B).[51] It also pays for such durable medical equipment as hospital beds, wheelchairs, breathing machines, and prosthetic devices and for up to three dialysis treatments a week for patients in renal failure.[52] Some medically necessary ambulance services are covered.[53]

Before 1990, Medicare covered few preventive services. Since then, Congress has added coverage of certain screening tests and preventive care such as mammography, Pap smears, pelvic and prostate exams, flu shots, colorectal screening, diabetes self-management training, and bone-mass measurements. The Medicare Modernization Act of 2003 (MMA), which mandated partial payment for outpatient prescription drugs, also expanded preventive services by offering advanced diabetes screening tests and various diagnostic tests for cardiovascular disease, as well as a comprehensive "Welcome to Medicare" physical exam for new enrollees. That said, gaps in prevention coverage continue.

### Prescription Drugs

Prescription drugs have become an increasingly important component of modern health care, particularly for the elderly, chronically ill, and people with disabilities.[54] Before 2004, Medicare paid only for drugs administered in hospitals and other institutional settings and for selected drugs administered in physicians' offices, primarily for cancer therapy. Nearly two-thirds of Medicare beneficiaries had drug coverage, usually private insurance or Medicaid. On the whole, private coverage was limited or expensive.[55]

The MMA changed this picture considerably, beginning with a transitional discount program implemented during 2004 and 2005 under Medicare's oversight. Private plans, pharmacy benefit managers, drug companies, and other entities offered beneficiaries cards that entitled them to discounts when they purchased drugs either at retail outlets that were part of the sponsor's network or through mail order.[56]

In January 2006 Medicare began its outpatient prescription drug benefit under a new Part D. Beneficiaries can join stand-alone prescription drug plans (PDPs) or secure drug coverage through their Medicare Advantage plans (MA-PDs).[57] The monthly PDP premium in 2008 averaged $40.02.[58] The standard benefit design for 2008 called for a $275 deductible, 25 percent coinsurance for expenditures between $275 and $2,510 in total drug costs, and 5 percent coinsurance for expenditures above a catastrophic threshold of $5,726.25.[59] The standard plan does not cover expenditures between $2,510 and $5,726.25—called the doughnut hole—although price discounts negotiated by participating plans are available in this range. Plans may offer other benefit designs as long as the value of coverage is not reduced and neither the deductible nor the threshold at which the 5 percent coinsurance begins is increased.[60] Plans can establish their own formularies of drugs to be covered, but each therapeutic class must include at least two compounds.[61] In general, payments for drug costs by third parties (such as a supplemental insurance plan) or outlays on off-formulary drugs do not count in determining whether the catastrophic threshold has been reached.[62]

DESIGN CONSTRAINTS. This bizarre benefit structure is the legislative response to four constraints. First, owing to the budget resolution of fiscal 2004, the ten-year cost of program benefits could not exceed $400 billion, which equaled about one-fourth of projected expenditures on prescription drugs for the Medicare population. Second, lawmakers made the political judgment that the benefit had to be voluntary—like Part B, but unlike the drug benefit in the ill-fated Medicare Catastrophic Coverage Act of 1988.[63] This political decision meant that the government had to heavily subsidize premiums to encourage voluntary enrollment. Third, the legislation could not limit its coverage to catastrophic coverage since such a limit would discourage enrollment by all except those with large drug expenditures, which would cause the entire program to collapse. Consequently, the bill provided a low deductible to attract those with modest expenditures.[64] Fourth, legislators decided to deeply subsidize low-income enrollees (see box 2-2). To meet these constraints, the legislation created a gap in the coverage—the doughnut hole.

ADMINISTRATION. Private plans are entirely responsible for administering the drug benefit. They are paid under a complex system that requires them to bear some financial risk. This design is intended to spur competition to keep drug prices, use, and premiums low (see box 2-3). Medicare also makes payments to employer- and union-sponsored retiree health plans that provide retiree coverage at least as generous as that provided by the standard benefit under Part D.[65]

## Coverage under Other Programs

Medicare's health care coverage is less generous than that of most private plans. As a result, most beneficiaries—91 percent in 2004—have additional coverage.[66] Some rely on retiree health policies, Medigap insurance, and Medicaid; others on Medicare Advantage.

Box 2-2. *Low-Income Subsidy Program for Part D*

Low-income Medicare beneficiaries can qualify for one of three levels of assistance for premiums and cost sharing for covered prescription drugs in Medicare. The poor who are eligible for both Medicare and Medicaid pay no premium for a plan with a premium at or below the regional average. They pay no deductible and co-payments of $1.05 to $3.10 for covered drugs in 2008. Other participants with incomes below 135 percent of the poverty threshold and limited assets also pay no premium for a plan with a premium at or below average. They pay no deductible and co-payments of $2.25 to $5.60 in 2008. Those with incomes below 150 percent of the poverty threshold and limited assets pay a sliding-scale premium, a $56 deductible, and 15 percent cost sharing for covered drugs below $5,726.25 in total spending in 2008 (all amounts indexed in subsequent years). The doughnut hole does not apply to participants in Medicare's low-income subsidy program.

## Employer Coverage

To attract and retain workers, some companies offer health benefits to retirees as well as active workers. These plans usually pay only for services covered by the company's plan but not by Medicare. They may also pay part or all of Medicare's cost sharing. Since 1995, employers have been curtailing retiree coverage, dropping benefits altogether, or requiring participating retirees to pay higher premiums.[67] These trends are a response, first, to fast-rising retiree health costs, which businesses are now straining to pay for. Second, under a 1990 regulation by the Financial Accounting Standards Board, companies must report on their balance sheets the present discounted value of the health benefits promised to retirees. This requirement has forced management and shareholders alike to face up to these liabilities—typically by reducing them. A similar accounting standard is now being phased in for public employees. Third, the Medicare drug benefit reduced the need for retiree coverage. Despite these pressures, employer-based plans remain the most common source of Medicare supplemental coverage.

## Medigap

Before 1990, private individual-market insurers offered Medicare beneficiaries a confusing array of supplemental plans at widely varying premiums.

Box 2-3. *How Medicare Pays Prescription Drug Plans*

Medicare pays for prescription drugs through direct subsidies to private plans, reinsurance, and risk corridors. Direct subsidies are based on a bidding process. PDPs and MA-PDs submit bids to Medicare that reflect the plan's expected costs of providing an average enrollee with the standard drug benefit. The direct subsidies paid to these plans by Medicare are based on these bids. Such payments are adjusted for enrollees' age, sex, health status, and, if applicable, participation in the low-income subsidy program and institutional status. Medicare also calculates premiums for each plan according to an MMA rule that enrollees (other than low-income subsidy enrollees) pay 25.5 percent of total program costs. However, enrollees must shoulder a larger percentage of the national average bid in order to pay 25.5 percent of total costs, as federal payments cover most costs above the catastrophic threshold (see below). For 2008 the percentage is about 35 percent, resulting in a national base beneficiary premium of $27.93.[1] Enrollees pay this amount plus or minus the difference between the selected plan's bid and the national average bid. Under this system, enrollees in effect pay for the full excess of a plan's bid over the national average and pay lower premiums if the bid is below the benchmark.

Medicare also pays PDPs and MA-PDs reinsurance if needed. Specifically, it finances 80 percent of drug expenditures that exceed the catastrophic threshold. In addition, the program makes extra payments to plans if their costs exceed, by certain margins, those assumed in their bid (called risk corridors). Conversely, if costs are significantly less than those assumed in a plan's bid, Medicare recoups money from the plan.[2] In general, Medicare's payments cover an estimated three-quarters of the average plan's costs for the standard benefit, plus subsidies to low-income enrollees.[3]

1. For a detailed description of Part D bid and beneficiary premium calculations, see Mark Merlis, *Medicare Payments and Beneficiary Costs for Prescription Drug Coverage* (Menlo Park, Calif.: Kaiser Family Foundation, 2007) (www.kff.org/medicare/upload/7620.pdf).
2. If the plan's total spending for standard drug benefits—net of rebates, administrative costs, and reinsurance payments—diverges from the target by 5 percent or more, the government shares the loss or gain. In the case of a 5–10 percent deviation, Medicare pays half of the loss or recoups half of the gain. If the plan departs from its target by more than 10 percent, Medicare absorbs 80 percent of the loss or keeps 80 percent of the gain. These risk corridors will remain in effect through 2011, after which the secretary of health and human services can set the risk corridors at no less than 5 percent.
3. MedPAC, *Medicare Payment Basics: Part D Payment System* (October 2007).

Comparing plans was exceedingly difficult. Some people ended up buying duplicate coverage or policies of little worth. In 1990 Congress asked the National Association of Insurance Commissioners (NAIC) to define a limited number of options for supplemental coverage that could be offered to Medicare participants. The NAIC came up with ten Medigap insurance packages that until 2006 were the only options available to Medicare beneficiaries participating in the individual insurance market.[68] Beginning in 2006, no new policies could include drug coverage, but two new benefit packages that cover catastrophic medical expenses became available.

The reforms of the 1990s helped to standardize benefits, increased the reliability of plans, and, in some cases, improved access to coverage. They required insurers offering Medigap policies to pay out at least a minimum portion of their premium income in benefits. They prohibited companies from denying coverage to Medicare participants who seek coverage during the first six months after they turn sixty-five or cease to be covered by an employer-sponsored retiree health plan, another Medigap plan, or a Medicare Advantage plan. They also banned premium variations based on an applicant's health risks. Insurers must set their premiums on a community-rated basis or according to participants' ages or the age when they first purchased insurance.[69] In 2004, 29 percent of the Medicare population was covered by Medigap.[70] Purchase of Medigap is most likely among those in rural areas, the elderly (as opposed to people with disabilities or patients with renal failure), the very old, the well-to-do, women, and those in relatively good health.[71]

### Medicaid

Poor Medicare enrollees may also qualify either for full Medicaid benefits (as so-called dual-eligibles) or for one of its Medicare Savings Programs. For dual-eligibles, Medicaid pays all Medicare premiums and cost sharing and covers nursing home care and some other services not covered by Medicare. Benefits and eligibility thresholds vary across the states.[72] In addition, four other programs exist for seniors who have low incomes and few assets but do not qualify for full Medicaid benefits. These Medicare Savings Programs provide full or partial assistance in paying for Medicare's Part A and B premiums and cost sharing (see box 2-4). As described earlier, beneficiaries may also qualify for the drug benefit's Medicare-administered low-income subsidy program, which eliminates or reduces premiums and cost sharing for Part D.

Box 2-4. *Dual-Eligibles, QMB, SLMB, QI, and QDWI*

In 2008 Medicaid provided assistance with Medicare's Part A and B premiums and cost sharing for 17.8 percent of beneficiaries. Of this group, 14.0 percent qualified for full Medicaid benefits as so-called dual-eligibles, and 3.8 percent received assistance through a Medicare Savings Program as qualified Medicare beneficiaries (QMBs), special low-income Medicare beneficiaries (SLMBs), qualified individuals (QIs), or qualified disabled and working individuals (QDWIs).[1] Dual-eligibles are covered primarily by Medicare but are also entitled to the full Medicaid benefit package, which acts as supplemental insurance to Medicare. The QMB program covers Medicare's Part A and B premiums and cost sharing for those whose incomes exceed their state's Medicaid threshold but fall below official federal poverty guidelines.[2] Under the SLMB program, Medicaid pays the Part B premiums of those with incomes at or above poverty but below 120 percent of federal guidelines. The QI program pays Medicare's Part B premium for individuals with incomes from 120 to 135 percent of poverty up to a cap. In addition, people with disabilities with incomes below 200 percent of poverty who returned to work and lost Part A benefits can regain them under the QDWI program.[3] Many who qualify for QMB and SLMB do not participate for one or more of several possible reasons: administrative complexity, the burden of the periodic eligibility determination, limited benefits, a lack of awareness that this assistance is available, cultural values of self-reliance, or the perceived stigma associated with welfare programs. Of those eligible for QMB and SLMB, only 33 percent and 13 percent participate, respectively.[4]

1. CMS, Part D Enrollment Data, *2008 Enrollment Information* (January 2008) (www.cms.hhs.gov/PrescriptionDrugCovGenIn).
2. Official 2008 federal poverty guidelines for the contiguous 48 states and the District of Columbia were $10,400 for individuals and $14,000 for couples.
3. The Medicare Savings Programs also impose an asset test of two times the basic asset test for the Supplemental Security Income program. The corresponding limits for 2008 were $4,000 for individuals and $6,000 for couples.
4. Congressional Budget Office, *A Detailed Description of CBO's Cost Estimate for the Medicare Prescription Drug Benefit* (July 2004), p. 29.

## Medicare Advantage

Before 1998, private plans that covered Medicare benefits received 95 percent of the local average per capita costs of Medicare, adjusted for simple risk measures. The rationale was that if plans could offer the same benefits at a 5 percent discount, the program would provide choice for beneficiaries as well as program savings. However, because MA enrollees were on average younger and healthier than those who remained in traditional Medicare, MA plans offered extra services (including prescription drugs), waived deductibles, and reduced cost sharing. Enrollment in MA plans grew 30 percent a year in the mid-1990s and reached 16 percent of Medicare beneficiaries in 1999.[73]

The Balanced Budget Act of 1997 reduced MA overpayments and began to phase in improved methods of risk-adjusting plan payments. Many plans dropped out of the program. Others stopped serving some areas or reduced supplemental coverage.[74] MA enrollment growth slowed in 1997 and then began to decline in 2000.[75]

In an effort to boost MA enrollment, Congress raised MA fees in 2003. Then in 2006 it launched a competitive payment system that requires MA plans to submit bids stating how much they will charge to offer an average Medicare beneficiary the Medicare benefit package (minus prescription drugs, which are paid for separately).[76] They get paid this bid, with an adjustment for the average expected cost of enrollees. If the bid is below the local average of bids, or "benchmark," plans must return most of the overpayment to beneficiaries through reduced premiums or enriched benefits. If the bid is above the benchmark, the excess amount is added to enrollees' premiums.

Most Medicare Advantage participants enroll in health maintenance organizations (HMOs) or some other type of managed care plan.[77] These plans typically concentrate in counties where capitation rates are high. In 1997 several new options were created. Private fee-for-service plans offer open access to all providers who accept the plan rates but may charge enrollees higher cost sharing for this access.[78] Enrollment in private fee-for-service plans has grown rapidly, especially in rural areas, because overpayments from Medicare have allowed such plans to reduce Medicare premiums and cost sharing, if not overall costs. The MMA also offers strong tax incentives for enrollees to open medical savings accounts (MSAs) and to buy high-deductible insurance. Despite these incentives, only nine such plans were being offered in 2008, with a combined enrollment of only 3,300.[79] The MMA also authorized "special needs" plans whose enrollment is limited to those with special needs, such as dual-eligibles, institutionalized individuals, and the people with disabilities.[80] Beginning in 2006, beneficiaries were given the additional option of enrolling in regional preferred provider organizations (PPOs).[81]

On average, Medicare Advantage plans in 2008 were paid 13 percent more than the cost of covering their enrollees under the fee-for-service delivery system—as much as 50 percent more in some areas. [82] These overpayments will boost Medicare spending by more than $150 billion in the decade from 2008 to 2017 and reduce the life of the Health Insurance trust fund by eighteen months.[83] The significant payment increase brought about by the MMA caused many MA plans to lower or eliminate their supplemental premiums and enrich their benefit packages. As a result, the proportion of Medicare participants enrolled in MA plans rose to 18 percent in 2007, surpassing the previous high of 16 percent in 1999.[84] By 2006 Medicare Advantage plans were available to all Medicare enrollees.[85] Projections indicate that 25 percent of Medicare beneficiaries will be enrolled in MA plans by 2013.[86]

## Financing Medicare

Still bearing the imprint of the legislative compromise that led to its enactment, Medicare finances its benefits through a combination of dedicated payroll taxes, general revenues, and individual premiums. All flow through two separate trust funds from which payments for Part A and Part B—as well as Parts C and D—services are made.

The principal source of revenue for Part A is a 2.9 percentage point payroll tax on all workers' earnings, half levied on workers, half on employers. In 2007 this tax supplied 86 percent of the Hospital Insurance trust fund's income.[87] The remainder comes from earmarked personal income tax revenues collected on a portion of the benefits received by high-income Social Security beneficiaries (4.7 percent), interest earnings on HI trust fund reserves (7.4 percent), and various other receipts.[88] Any excess of income over benefits and administrative costs is added to the HI trust fund reserves. These reserves totaled $326 billion at the end of 2007.[89] Premiums of Part B enrollees, which are set to cover about one-quarter of Part B program costs, flow into the Supplementary Medical Insurance trust fund. Premiums are deducted automatically from participants' Social Security benefits. By law, general treasury revenues cover most of the balance of Part B spending.[90]

Part D drug benefits are also financed by a combination of general revenues and premiums paid by those who elect Part D coverage. In addition, the Part D account in the SMI trust fund receives payments from the states that approximate a percentage of the savings they are deemed to have realized when dual-eligibles (whose drug benefits had been covered by Medicaid) were moved to Medicare by the MMA. General revenues also subsidize beneficiaries who enroll in its low-income subsidy program. The total government subsidy for the Medicare population in general is equal to nearly 75 percent of program costs for basic drug coverage.

According to estimates released in 2008, the Hospital Insurance program is adequately funded until early 2019.[91] However, outlays of Part A are projected to exceed revenues in 2010, despite its sizable reserves. By law, Supplemental Medical Insurance is always adequately funded, as it has an automatic tap on general revenues to cover outlays in excess of premium income. The same is true of Part D. Although Medicare is entitled by legislation to draw on general revenues for most of the costs of Parts B and D, Congress feared that the general revenue burden was becoming excessive and in the MMA called on Medicare actuaries to report when general revenues are expected to cover more than 45 percent of Medicare's total outlays within a seven-year projection period. If such determinations are made in two consecutive reports, the president is required to present to Congress proposals on how to bring the fraction down below the threshold. Congress must consider any such proposal under special rules but is not required to reduce the fraction below 45 percent. The purpose of this provision is to focus attention on the budgetary impact of Medicare and, possibly, to reduce Medicare spending or increase its dedicated taxes.[92]

## Summary

Thanks to Medicare, a larger fraction of the elderly than of any other age group is insured. Compared with those insured by employer-sponsored plans, Medicare beneficiaries are more likely to rate their health insurance as excellent and less likely to report negative insurance experiences or to say they could not get health care because of cost. Furthermore, they are more likely than those with private insurance to report being very satisfied with the care they received.[93] Despite this creditable record, the program still falls short in benefit coverage, quality, and cost. The next chapter examines those shortcomings in detail, as a foundation for considering how best to reform the system.

# 3
## Goals, Performance, and Options for Medicare

Medicare is hugely popular with both the public and policymakers. It provides nearly all people aged sixty-five or older and those with certain disabilities with health insurance that many would otherwise find costly or unavailable.[1] It covers most medical costs of its elderly enrollees. It offers beneficiaries more choice of providers than do most health plans serving workers and their dependents. In addition, Medicare is an important source of employment, providing billions of dollars in income to hospitals, doctors, home health agencies, nursing homes, drug companies and pharmacies, medical device manufacturers, and other providers in every congressional district.

Notwithstanding its popularity and positive results, Medicare suffers from serious flaws and faces daunting challenges. Its benefits have gaps, especially for people with mental illnesses or those who need long-term care. Its focus on quality has been weak. And it is on track to impose ever-growing burdens on taxpayers. Projected Hospital Insurance (HI) outlays, for example, will likely exceed earmarked payroll and income taxes in the near future.[2] Demands on general revenues to pay for Supplemental Medical Insurance (SMI) threaten severe federal budget deficits unless taxes are greatly increased. The rapid growth of health spending in public programs accounts entirely for the large projected budget deficits (table 3-1).[3]

Table 3-1. *Projected "Primary" Budget Deficit (−) or Surplus (+): Including and Excluding Medicare and Medicaid, Selected Years, 2007–80*[a]
Percent of GDP

| | Projected deficit or surplus | |
|---|---|---|
| Year | Including all expenditures and revenues | Excluding Medicare and Medicaid and associated revenues |
| 2007 (actual) | +0.8 | +0.7 |
| 2010 | +0.7 | +0.9 |
| 2020 | +0.0 | +1.6 |
| 2030 | −2.9 | +0.9 |
| 2040 | −5.0 | +0.8 |
| 2050 | −6.3 | +1.4 |
| 2060 | −7.9 | +1.7 |
| 2070 | −9.5 | +2.2 |
| 2080 | −11.2 | +2.6 |

Source: Henry Aaron's calculations based on unpublished data underlying the Congressional Budget Office (CBO), *The Long-Term Budget Outlook* (December 2007); CBO, "Update of CBO's Economic Forecast," Letter to the Honorable Kent Conrad (Washington, February 15, 2008); FHI Board of Trustees, *2008 Annual Report.* The data combine CBO's extended-baseline scenario for expenditures (adheres most closely to current law and assumes physician payment cuts as scheduled under the SGR) and its alternative fiscal scenario for revenues (assumes that none of the changes to tax law scheduled after 2007 will take effect and that the AMT will be indexed to inflation).

a. The "primary" deficit or surplus is defined as all government spending, excluding interest on the debt, less all government revenue. Projected deficit excluding Medicare, Medicaid, and associated revenues is computed as follows: (1) projected Medicare and Medicaid spending are subtracted from CBO's projection of total long-term spending, excluding interest payments (following CBO's convention, beneficiary premiums are included in outlays as offsetting receipts); (2) from projected total revenues the following items are subtracted: projected Medicare payroll taxes, revenues from taxation of certain Social Security benefits that are transferred to Medicare, Part D "clawback" payments by states, and general revenues used to finance Medicare and Medicaid in 2007. The "projected deficit, excluding Medicare and Medicaid and associated revenues" is the difference between (1) and (2). It excludes from the projected deficit the anticipated increase in general revenues that will be needed to support Medicare and Medicaid if health care spending per beneficiary continues to outpace income growth by amounts as projected by the CBO in *The Long-Term Outlook for Health Care Spending* (November 2007).

Some shortcomings are structural. For one, the distinction between hospital care (Part A) and physician services (Part B) laid out when Medicare was created is now regarded as artificial. For another, the drug benefit is administered separately. Equally troubling, Medicare has failed to adapt quickly to the scientific advances that are remaking health care and the mode of its delivery. Other shortcomings—for instance, Medicare's failure to promote coordinated care for those with multiple illnesses—are common to private insurance as well. Still others are rooted in the difficulties inherent in designing and administering a uniform national program capable of providing thousands of locally produced and delivered services in hundreds of markets to a heterogeneous clientele of 44 million.

Perhaps the first question to ask in assessing program performance is how well or how poorly the program meets its goals, which are to ensure beneficiaries access to high-quality health care produced in an affordable manner. These three goals—access, quality, and cost control—are interwoven yet may conflict with one another.

## Ensuring Access

Access means that a person who needs health care can afford it and find it. Clearly, a person without insurance coverage may not be able to afford health services, but insurance will be of limited value if cost sharing is so high that care remains unaffordable. Access will still be limited if providers are excluded from the insurance network in order to wrest price discounts from those who are included in the network. At the same time, very low payment rates may discourage providers from serving covered patients and thus further impede access. In addition, services may be inaccessible when care is needed, a common problem in rural and underserved urban areas. All in all, access to care is a large concern in Medicare because many of its beneficiaries have low income and high health care needs.

### Financial Access

Medicare and supplemental coverage together do quite well in ensuring beneficiaries' financial access to care. Although the Medicare benefit package in some important respects remains inferior to the health plans in which most working Americans and their dependents are enrolled, it covers most standard forms of medical care. Physician visits, lab tests, and home health are covered without limit. But hospital stays are subject to the complex limits and cost sharing described in chapter 2. Skilled nursing facility (SNF) stays are limited to 100 days. Medicare still does not cover periodic health exams after initial enrollment for asymptomatic individuals or services related to vision, hearing impairment, or dental care.[4]

Medicare's cost sharing, adopted piecemeal as various benefits were added or modified over the years, follows no logical pattern. The cost-sharing rate for physician and most outpatient services is 20 percent of fees

Medicare has set.[5] The inpatient hospital deductible is much higher than under most private plans.[6] Daily co-payments begin on the sixty-first day of an episode. Beneficiaries must pay more for outpatient hospital and SNF services than is typical of employer-sponsored policies for workers.[7] Deductibles and coinsurance are waived for some preventive services but not for others. One deductible is ghoulish: beneficiaries must pay for the first three pints of blood they receive in a year. On the other hand, home health visits and laboratory tests, for example, have no coinsurance or co-payments. Medicare lacks a limit on total out-of-pocket expenses, a feature of roughly 70 percent of workers' plans.[8] Such a benefit protects beneficiaries from the catastrophic liabilities that can arise from a serious illness or a chronic condition.

Thus the burden of Medicare cost sharing and deductibles depends on the luck of the draw. For example, frail elderly beneficiaries in need of long-term care bear no cost if services are provided through the home health benefit but could pay more than half the cost of care if they are delivered in a nursing home.

Overall, Medicare beneficiaries report high financial access to care. In 2005 fewer than 8 percent of noninstitutionalized beneficiaries said they delayed health care because of cost. Seniors were only three-fifths as likely as people aged fifty to sixty-four to report they had failed to obtain health care because of cost.[9]

Reform of deductibles and other cost sharing merits high priority in any proposed Medicare reform. Some cost sharing is essential to holding down burdens on taxpayers and preserving some cost sensitivity. Therefore most beneficiaries should face some charges for the health insurance they receive and the services they use. But low-income beneficiaries should be shielded from such costs, either through a separate assistance program, such as today's Medicaid, or through a means-tested mechanism incorporated into Medicare similar to the low-income subsidy program for the drug benefit. Furthermore, there should be a limit on out-of-pocket health spending for all enrollees, such as the one included in the Medicare drug benefit.

### Physical Access

Financial access is meaningful only if one can find and get to a physician who accepts Medicare patients or a hospital within reach. Medicare passes this test because of several specific policies. Nearly all health care providers in the country see Medicare enrollees.[10] Any licensed provider may receive payment for covered services, without the filters that some private insurers use to reduce cost and improve quality. Medicare rules have led most physicians either to forgo "balance billing" or to accept limits on how much they can charge beneficiaries in addition to Medicare's payment. These rules discourage most physicians from specializing in "diseases of the rich," catering only to beneficiaries who can afford high rates. Medicare has also dedicated extra payments to providers in rural and underserved communities. Where physical access to care is limited—as in sparsely populated rural areas or poor urban neighborhoods—the problem is not of Medicare's making. Indeed, many rural providers could not maintain their practices without revenue from Medicare. Medicare beneficiaries themselves report high levels of physical access to care. In 2005 only 4 percent of beneficiaries were dissatisfied with the ease of access to health care.[11]

A serious question for any reform plan, particularly one that eliminates Medicare's current payment systems, is whether and how to preserve hospitals, laboratories, and other medical facilities in thinly settled areas. Another important consideration is whether any changes will affect Medicare's open access to providers.

## Promoting Quality and Satisfaction

"High-quality" health care is both difficult to define and prone to controversy. No single measure can capture its many dimensions. The federal government, for example, tracks over forty core measures in its congressionally mandated *National Health Care Quality Report*. For many practitioners judged to be below standards others have set, the subject is a sensitive one.[12] The Institute of Medicine defines quality as "the degree to which health services for individuals and populations increase the likelihood of desired health outcomes and are consistent with current professional knowledge."[13] Others focus more on the degree to which health services are able to avoid three cardinal mistakes: overuse, underuse, and misuse.[14] Another factor increasingly relevant to quality is cost. When resources are limited, procedures that offer low value per dollar of cost deny resources to other patients. Excessive cost, often from provider inefficiency or administrative waste, can also be a problem. Excessive deductibles can discourage needed care, and low cost sharing can encourage demand for care of marginal value.

By almost any measure, the quality of care in the United States is uneven and low in relation to what people pay for it. As research has revealed, patients on average receive barely more than half of recommended care for the conditions they have.[15] This dismal pattern applies broadly to old and young; poor and rich; whites, blacks, and Hispanics; men and women; and Medicare beneficiaries. In 2004 more than 6 percent of Medicare beneficiaries hospitalized for surgery developed preventable postoperative complications such as pneumonia, urinary tract infection, and blood clots in the legs, and only 58 percent were given antibiotics at medically indicated times.[16] About one in twenty hospitalized Medicare beneficiaries experienced an adverse drug event, a rate nearly two times greater than that for patients with private health insurance.[17] Between 1998 and 2006, adverse events experienced by hospitalized Medicare patients increased in five of the nine most common categories.[18] In addition, one-third of seriously ill U.S. patients reported a medical mistake, medication error, or lab test error in 2005, a rate over 50 percent higher than that in Germany and the United Kingdom.[19]

With the growing realization that a wide gap separates actual from optimal practice, private insurers and employers have begun to invest time and money to improve the quality of care. In extreme cases, they refuse to pay those who do not meet minimum standards. Some companies even inform employees about the relative performance of insurance plans and of covered physicians and hospitals.[20] A few pay increased fees to high-quality providers. Most health maintenance organizations (including Medicare Advantage plans) have their performance evaluated on the basis of the Health Care Effectiveness Data and Information Set (HEDIS) devised by the National Committee for Quality Assurance (NCQA).[21] Some health plans evaluate new technologies for cost and efficacy and use this information to decide what to cover and to educate providers.

### Efforts to Improve Quality

A major obstacle to quality improvement is that most medical procedures, old and new, have not been evaluated for comparative cost- and clinical effectiveness. In the absence of such information, it has been difficult to establish evidence-based medical standards for what constitutes high-quality care. Even if the necessary evidence had been available in the 1960s, Medicare would have had to tread lightly because many feared that the program might lure the nation into "socialized" medicine. No program could second-guess physicians if it was to be politically acceptable. The Medicare law bluntly declared: "Nothing in this title shall be construed to authorize any Federal officer or employee to exercise any supervision or control over the practice of medicine."[22] Furthermore, Medicare had to pay "any willing provider"—that is, any licensed doctor, hospital, or clinic that agreed to abide by Medicare's rules, accept its payment rates, and serve Medicare beneficiaries.

This is not to say that no attempts were made to monitor quality. Various efforts were launched early in the program to review professional standards, peer practice, and experimental medical care. They made little headway, however, because they were voluntary and the information necessary to make sound quality judgments was unavailable.[23] In 1982 Congress created the Medicare Quality Improvement Program, which subjected case records to peer review and other forms of retrospective management by contracted physician-run groups (now called quality improvement organizations, or QIOs). In the 1990s the program began trying to measure quality but employed crude measures of outcome. In recent years, it has turned to measures based on processes of care, but critics think this approach is too narrow and removed from the kind of technical assistance needed to improve quality.[24]

Policy is changing, as private and public payers alike now recognize that U.S. health providers do not consistently deliver high-quality care. Experts have come to believe that quality will improve if the manner of delivering health care is changed through greater use of health information technology and collaboration among the progressively narrower specializations involved in delivering modern health care.[25]

Medicare currently bases payments on procedures and inputs. Some analysts would instead link payments to outcomes or to specific services that research has shown to be beneficial and cost-effective; this is the so-called pay-for-performance (P4P) approach. Medicare is undertaking several pilot programs to test payment of hospitals and physicians based on objective measures of medical practice. It is also carrying out demonstrations of coordinated care for patients with chronic conditions, such as diabetes, congestive heart failure, and end-stage renal disease.[26] In 2007 Medicare announced that it would no longer pay for care that generates errors that should never happen—such as amputation of the wrong limb.

### Innovation

Boosting health care quality requires new and improved techniques, technology, and pharmaceuticals. Medicare has been repeatedly criticized for moving too slowly to cover such advances. Some of this tardiness stems from the need for congressional approval of major changes, such as the addition of a drug benefit. And some relates to the regulatory process for determining coverage. The Social Security Act requires Medicare to pay for all medical care that is "reasonable and necessary."[27] Realistically, this requirement is unachievable. Necessary limits on coverage prevent payment for some medically necessary care. And many traditional therapies have never been rigorously evaluated. Many never will be, because denying therapies widely *believed* to be effective, even if untested, is considered unethical.

Some Medicare coverage decisions are made nationally by the Centers for Medicare and Medicaid Services (CMS). Most are made locally by the medical directors of the contractors responsible for Medicare claims processing, review, and adjudication in each region of the country. As a result, new technologies may be approved in one place but not in another. CMS decisions generally require an independent assessment of safety and effectiveness.[28] Medicare has recently tried to speed up the adoption of new technologies without compromising safety.[29]

Medicare is not alone in being slow to promote high-value services. The U.S. record in this regard is substandard. Other nations have established and sustained publicly funded agencies to evaluate new medical technologies for cost-effectiveness.[30] In the United States, unfortunately, Congress has killed or weakened such agencies when they issued findings that powerful interests found objectionable.[31]

Whether patients have suffered on balance because of Medicare's cautious approval policy is unclear. Delay is prudent, especially for high-risk populations, when new procedures are propelled by ill-informed enthusiasm or commercial motives rather than medical evidence. In one such case, private insurers rushed to cover a costly treatment for breast cancer patients—high-dose chemotherapy followed by autologous bone-marrow transplants—that clinical trials eventually revealed to be ineffective. On the whole, however, Medicare's incentive structure is more supportive of innovation than is often portrayed. Flat, prospective payments to hospitals and many other providers for a bundle of services encourages adoption of new devices and procedures and methods that lower the cost of achieving a given medical outcome as soon as they are approved by the Food and Drug Administration or relevant regulatory body.

### Satisfaction

Consumer satisfaction is one component of high-quality health care. On this score, Medicare ranks high. In a Commonwealth Fund survey, elderly Medicare patients ranked their care more favorably than did nonelderly patients covered by private insurance (table 3-2).[32] The role of

Table 3-2. *Satisfaction with Health Insurance, 2001*[a]

Percent of respondents

| Response | Medicare, elderly, ≥ age 65 | Medicare, disabled, < age 65 | Privately insured, aged 19–64 |
|---|---|---|---|
| Health insurance very good or excellent | 66 | 39 | 54 |
| Very satisfied with health care | 62 | 46 | 51 |
| Very confident in future ability to get care | 50 | 36 | 37 |
| Never had coverage problem with current insurance | 57 | 36 | 39 |
| Did not go without medical care in past year because of cost | 82 | 58 | 78 |

Source: Karen Davis and others, "Medicare versus Private Insurance: Rhetoric and Reality," *Health Affairs*, Web Exclusive (October 9, 2002): W311–24.

a. Based on data from the Commonwealth Fund's 2001 *Survey of Health Insurance*, which was conducted by Princeton Survey Research Associates from April 27 through July 29, 2001. The interviews included 1,878 privately insured adults aged nineteen to sixty-four, 584 Medicare beneficiaries aged sixty-five and older, and 157 disabled Medicare beneficiaries aged sixty-four and younger. As of April 2008, no follow-up survey had been published. Comparable surveys with separate elderly and nonelderly samples were published, however, with results similar to those presented here.

patient satisfaction is clearly important in a public program that is subject to political review. Unfortunately, that satisfaction does not correlate with the technical quality of the care provided, at least among vulnerable elderly patients.[33]

### Quality and Medicare Reform

How Medicare reform affects the quality of care in all its dimensions should be a prime consideration in assessing reform proposals. As the largest single payer for health care, Medicare has the potential—largely unexploited—to spur administrative innovation, inform consumers, evaluate new medical technologies, and improve the organization of medical practice. How reform affects the quality of health care for Medicare beneficiaries will affect the well-being of all Americans.

One of the government's most important functions is to shape institutions that influence the quality of life of its citizens. To this end, governments can create and disseminate relevant information, which is precisely what they do best. In chapter 4 we describe procedures under which the "social insurance" version of Medicare could play a leading role in evaluating medical services and technologies to generate information on the cost of improving the quality of life and extending its duration. But other public agencies could perform similar functions if Medicare is reformed along the lines outlined in chapters 5 or 6.

## Controlling Costs

The primary political reason for the urgency of Medicare reform is the projected gap between the growth of Medicare outlays and revenues (table 3-3). If the growth of Medicare and Medicaid spending does not slow, record tax increases will be necessary over the coming decades to sustain existing coverage. But predictions of rapid spending growth are not new. Since enactment, Medicare has claimed a progressively larger share of aggregate federal spending and national income. This trend had little to do with enrollment growth. Whereas the proportion of the U.S. population receiving Medicare increased only 25 percent—from 12 percent in 1975 to 15 percent in 2007—the share of gross domestic product (GDP) devoted to Medicare more than doubled.[34] Annual growth of real per capita spending on all health care outpaced income growth by an average of 2.1 percentage points from 1975 to 2005. Medicare spending per beneficiary grew even faster at 2.4 percentage points.[35]

Medicare's cost growth has roughly paralleled that of private health spending, but if levels are examined, Medicare generally pays less for services than do private insurers.[36] Medicare's payments to physicians average about 81 percent of the rates paid by private insurers; hospital rates follow a similar pattern.[37] Medicare also has lower administrative costs than private insurers: 3–5 percent of outlays for Medicare versus 9–30 percent for private insurers.[38] High use by its comparatively old and sick population partly offset Medicare's lower prices and administrative costs. Its payment methods also require constant calibration and occasional overhaul. But Medicare's cost control has not lagged far behind that of other health insurers.

However, a *comparatively* good performance may not be good enough. There is no reason to expect the gap between the growth of income and health care spending to narrow in the near future.[39] Furthermore, the proportion of the U.S. population receiving Medicare is expected to grow from 15 percent in 2007 to 22 percent in 2030. The interaction of these two forces—rising per capita health care spending and growing enrollment—accounts for the huge projected increase in Medicare spending, as well as the likelihood of a debate over ways to address it.[40]

Table 3-3. *Projected Medicare Fiscal Gap, Selected Years, 2007–80*
Percent of GDP

| Year | Payroll taxes | Premiums[a] | Other earmarked revenues[b] | General revenue | Total income[c] | Total outlays | Fiscal gap (HI income shortfall plus SMI general revenue contribution)[d] |
|---|---|---|---|---|---|---|---|
| 2007 (actual) | 1.4 | 0.4 | 0.1 | 1.3 | 3.2 | 3.1 | 1.2 |
| 2010 | 1.4 | 0.4 | 0.2 | 1.2 | 3.1 | 3.4 | 1.4 |
| 2020 | 1.4 | 0.5 | 0.2 | 1.9 | 4.0 | 4.4 | 2.3 |
| 2030 | 1.3 | 0.8 | 0.3 | 2.7 | 5.1 | 6.3 | 3.8 |
| 2040 | 1.3 | 0.9 | 0.3 | 3.2 | 5.8 | 7.6 | 5.0 |
| 2050 | 1.3 | 1.0 | 0.3 | 3.6 | 6.2 | 8.4 | 5.7 |
| 2060 | 1.3 | 1.2 | 0.4 | 3.9 | 6.7 | 9.2 | 6.4 |
| 2070 | 1.2 | 1.3 | 0.4 | 4.2 | 7.1 | 10.0 | 7.1 |
| 2080 | 1.2 | 1.4 | 0.4 | 4.5 | 7.5 | 10.7 | 7.7 |

Source: Unpublished data underlying the FHI Board of Trustees, *2008 Annual Report*. Supplied by CMS, Office of the Actuary (April 2, 2008).

a. Includes premium revenue from HI and both accounts in the SMI trust fund.

b. Includes revenues from taxation of certain Social Security benefits that are transferred to Medicare and Part D "clawback" payments by states.

c. Excludes interest earnings on invested HI and SMI trust fund assets. Unlike CBO projections, which include beneficiary premiums as offsetting receipts in outlays, the Medicare trustees' figures include this series as income.

d. Calculated as the sum of total outlays minus total income and general revenue income. For further details on this method, see note 52 in the text.

There are five main ways to deal with this challenge: control prices, reduce use, improve health care efficiency, scale back coverage, and raise revenue. The first three options would reduce the overall cost of health care for a given population and set of benefits. The reforms described in this book combine these options in different ways to achieve Medicare's goals of good access, high quality, and cost containment. The fourth and fifth options—scaling back coverage (for example, by reducing benefits or raising the age of eligibility for Medicare) and raising revenue—would close Medicare's financing gap but would do so in part by shifting costs to other insurers, beneficiaries, or taxpayers. Some of these changes will be necessary to solve Medicare's long-run challenges. We mention them briefly in this chapter, but they are not a focal point of this book.

## Limiting Prices

Total spending depends on how much care is rendered and how much each unit of service costs. Under traditional Medicare, most prices are determined through legislation and regulation. Medicare Advantage and the Part D drug program, in contrast, pay private plans fixed, risk-adjusted payments per enrollee to deliver services. These plans, in turn, determine prices. The program has been experimenting and, in limited cases, adopting competitive bidding to pay for certain services like durable medical equipment. Yet most Medicare spending is for services paid for through service-specific payment systems.

Medicare's payment policies have been revised periodically in an attempt to slow the growth of spending. The extent to which these efforts have succeeded is widely debated. Many health care providers argue that Medicare pays too little to cover costs and that its rules are arbitrary and too complex. (See appendix D for the current methods of price setting.) It is important to keep in mind that some administrative entity, private or public, must perform these functions. The policy debate concerns whether these functions are likely to be performed best privately or publicly.

Setting prices for physicians' services illustrates a larger class of problems: how to prevent sellers from unreasonably boosting prices when the ultimate buyer—the patient—is insured and, hence, relatively indifferent to cost. Although the resource-based relative value scale (RBRVS) and sustainable growth rate (SGR) systems have idiosyncratic flaws, no administered price regime can avoid similar complexity, controversy, and error. With control only over prices, federal policymakers can influence the quantity or character of services that physicians and hospitals provide only indirectly. Medicare reform can shift the locus of these problems. It cannot eliminate them. As noted earlier, the practical question is whether private or public regulators will secure better "value for money" for taxpayers, who support most of the cost of Medicare, and for patients, who receive Medicare services.

Ultimately, Congress must approve virtually every major cost-containment policy. Some argue that the growing power of particular interests in Medicare policy has precluded effective cost containment. Nonetheless, budget pressures along with concerns about Medicare's financial imbalance have led to almost annual changes to Medicare law, many of which have lowered its expenditures.

Redesigning the program would change political pressures for and against Medicare cost containment but not eliminate them. Under the premium support system described in chapter 5, beneficiaries would receive flat payments that they could use to buy insurance. But the level of these payments would likely remain the subject of intense debate. The interest of physician groups in the SGR system would be eliminated under consumer-directed Medicare. But providers would remain anxious to shape the legal definition of what constitutes an acceptable insurance plan to maintain demand for their services. The current system relies so heavily on specific regulations and on administered prices that it provides peculiarly favorable terrain for political lobbying. This would not change under a revised social insurance model.

Inaccurate billing and possible fraud are problems whenever an insurer pays for specific services. Were the services actually provided? Was the service the one listed on the invoice? This problem is acute when the service is as hard to classify as many medical services are. It has long been rumored that physicians and hospitals used this ambiguity to upgrade the complexity of services for which they billed—referred to as "DRG creep." During the 1990s, there were widespread reports of error and outright fraud in billing by hospitals, physicians, and other providers.

In response, Congress beefed up law enforcement in 1996. The Health Insurance Portability and Accountability Act (HIPAA) facilitated prosecutions under the False Claims Act, a law enacted during the Civil War to combat fraud by defense contractors. HIPAA also specified a new class of crimes called health care fraud. Criminal practices include billing for Medicare services that are not medically necessary. Even billing for an otherwise legitimate service under the wrong category became an indictable offense. HIPAA also created a new, well-funded Health Care Fraud and Abuse Control Program. Fines from successful cases returned an estimated $10.4 billion to the Medicare Hospital Insurance trust fund between 1997 and 2006.[41] Such litigation has helped create a hostile adversarial atmosphere between Medicare and providers.

### Limiting Use

Even if Medicare pays less per unit of service than other insurers do, some critics claim that fee-for-service payment promotes the overuse of care, inflating program cost. Physicians earn income from serving patients. They usually have no financial incentive to limit care even if it promises little benefit.[42] Supplemental policies that fully cover deductibles and cost sharing exacerbate this problem by insulating patients from costs at the time of care that might cause them to limit use. By reducing patients' sensitivity to price, insurance also mutes the incentive for physicians and other providers to hold down cost. Every health care system must grapple with the problems created by the relative indifference to total cost of well-insured patients and those who supply services.

The enormous variation in service use under Medicare across geographical areas raises some troubling questions. In 2003 Medicare reimbursements per beneficiary ranged from $4,520 in Salem, Oregon, to $11,422 in Miami, Florida.[43] Some variability is to be expected because the incidence of illnesses varies. But variability of practice habits contributes even more to differences among treatments and in expenditures. Those interventions for which there is little medical discretion, such as hospital admission for hip fractures, vary far less than do interventions whose medical value is subject to considerable controversy, such as back surgery.[44] If heavy use of discretionary procedures led to superior health outcomes, one might worry about their cost but not their efficacy. In fact, the high use of costly medical procedures is not always associated with superior outcomes.[45] Victims of heart attacks survive longer in communities that make heavy use of low-cost forms of care than in communities that most intensively use costly methods. Furthermore, per capita Medicare spending and survival in the year following a heart attack are negatively related. The cost of treating heart attacks, which had risen, along with survival rates, from 1985 to 1995, continued to increase over the next seven years with no further improvement in survival.

Several experiments are under way to determine whether coordination of care in complex cases can improve outcomes and save money. Medical professionals expect both gains to be realized. Unfortunately, with regard to one major experiment, these hopes have been fleeting. In their final four-year review, participating sites within the Medicare Coordinated Care Demonstration were found to have improved some aspects of quality of care but achieved no cost savings in doing so.[46]

### Improving Health Care Efficiency

The evidence on whether Medicare is an efficient purchaser is conflicting. A pricing demonstration in two sites revealed that, on average, Medicare paid more than 20 percent above market rates for certain types of durable medical equipment.[47] The Veterans Health Administration, which purchases medical supplies competitively, often pays prices well below those set by Medicare. Research suggests that Medicare could save money by bargaining with suppliers and providers over price, but it is also consistent with the view that private insurers might perform better than Medicare does now. In other situations, Medicare successfully exercises its market power. In some metropolitan areas, for example, Medicare's payments to physicians are much lower than those of the average private payer.[48] Because of Medicare's dominant market position and social importance, providers cannot readily turn their backs on the program.[49]

Improving administrative efficiency can also lower cost. On this dimension, Medicare scores well. Its billing systems are electronic. Its ratio of administrative staff to beneficiaries is lower than that of private insurers. It incurs no marketing costs. It need not maintain insurance reserves, produce a profit margin, or incur other operating expenses that are necessary for private insurers. Ironically, Medicare may be spending too little on administrative costs. Increased investment in managing new delivery system arrangements and review of high-cost cases, for example, could yield lower health spending and improve quality. Medicare has also failed to spearhead the move toward a fully integrated electronic medical record, a step that would improve both efficiency and quality.

## Meeting the Financial Challenge

Few Medicare beneficiaries—past or current—have paid enough, directly or through their employers, to cover the actuarial cost of the insurance they receive. Even future retirees, who will have paid higher taxes for more years than current retirees have, will receive benefits worth more than the taxes they and their employers have paid, because the rapid proliferation of new therapeutic and diagnostic procedures promises a continued increase in the cost of care per patient. As a result, active workers will continue to subsidize current retirees if Medicare coverage and financial protection remain comparable to the insurance of active workers and if premiums and cost sharing are not markedly increased.[50] Furthermore, no plausible increase in the age of eligibility for benefits could prevent an increase in the ratio of beneficiaries to active workers through about 2035 as baby-boomers age.

Because taxes in the long run must equal benefits, a continuation of current benefits and eligibility without large tax increases on active workers is mathematically impossible. If today's workers were required both to save enough to prepay their own future health care and to support care for current beneficiaries, they would pay far more in taxes than the value of the benefits they will eventually receive.

## The Gap

Projections of the CMS chief actuary indicate that Medicare expenditures will double as a share of GDP between 2007 and 2030 and more than triple by 2065.[51] The projected gap between outlays and revenues (measured as the HI income shortfall plus the general revenue contribution to the SMI program) widens from 1.2 percent of GDP in 2007 to 7.7 in 2080 (table 3-3).[52] By comparison, total personal income tax revenues in 2007 equaled 8.6 percent of GDP.[53] This projection is based on the assumption that the growth of Medicare spending per beneficiary will exceed the growth of per capita income by 1 percentage point, a difference that is well below the historical average. If the growth of health care spending per beneficiary exceeds the growth of per capita income by 2.4 percentage points a year, the actual average rate from 1975 to 2005, Medicare spending will rise from 3 percent of GDP in 2007 to 25 percent in 2080 (table 3-4). The historical disparity between the growth of health care spending and income will not shrink unless policy is changed or the advance of medical technology slows.[54]

## Closing the Gap

Reducing the cost of current coverage alone will not suffice to prevent Medicare spending from claiming a growing share of general revenues. Beyond reducing the per capita cost of Medicare's current benefits, policymakers could close the fiscal gap either by reducing coverage or by raising taxes, premiums, or cost sharing. Table 3-5 includes a menu of such measures, each of which would close the gap by 1 percent of GDP in 2030.[55] Because the projected gap will greatly exceed one percentage point, several "doses" of the changes shown in table 3-5, as well as measures to curtail the cost of current benefits, will be needed to prevent health care spending from increasing the budget deficit.

RAISE THE AGE OF ELIGIBILITY. To reduce Medicare spending by 1 percent of GDP in 2030, the age of eligibility for the elderly would have to increase from sixty-five to sixty-nine. The savings from raising the age of initial eligibility are surprisingly small because the young elderly are healthier than older and disabled Medicare beneficiaries.[56]

Table 3-4. *Projected Medicare Spending under Different Assumptions of Excess Cost Growth, Selected Years, 2010–80*[a]

Percent of GDP

| Year | No excess cost growth[b] | 1 percentage point[c] | CBO extended baseline, 1.8 percentage ponits[d] | CBO alternative fiscal (baseline + physician payments indexed for inflation)[e] | Historical average excess cost growth, 2.4 percentage points[f] |
|---|---|---|---|---|---|
| 2010 | 3.2 | 3.2 | 3.2 | 3.4 | 3.3 |
| 2020 | 3.9 | 4.3 | 4.4 | 4.7 | 4.4 |
| 2030 | 4.6 | 5.7 | 6.5 | 6.9 | 6.7 |
| 2040 | 4.9 | 6.8 | 8.4 | 9.0 | 9.1 |
| 2050 | 5.0 | 7.6 | 10.3 | 10.9 | 11.7 |
| 2060 | 5.2 | 8.5 | 12.2 | 13.0 | 15.1 |
| 2070 | 5.3 | 9.7 | 14.4 | 15.3 | 19.5 |
| 2080 | 5.4 | 10.9 | 16.6 | 17.7 | 25.3 |

Source: Unpublished data underlying CBO, *The Long-Term Outlook for Health Care Spending.*

a. Excess cost growth refers to the number of percentage points by which the growth of spending on Medicare per beneficiary exceeds the growth of real GDP per capita. Following the Medicare trustees' convention, Medicare spending is projected gross of the premiums paid by beneficiaries.

b. With no excess cost growth, the growth in health care costs would result solely from changes in the size and demographic composition of the enrolled populations.

c. A 1 percent excess cost growth is consistent with the Medicare trustees' intermediate scenario for their long-range forecasts, where they assume an average of this excess rate from the twenty-fifth to the seventy-fifth year of the projection period.

d. CBO assumes that excess cost growth through 2018 for Medicare will equal historical averages. CBO's projection methodology for excess cost growth from 2019 through 2082 assumes that (1) even in the absence of changes in federal law, spending growth will slow eventually as health care expenditures continue to rise and displace increasing amounts of consumption of goods and services besides health care, and (2) steps taken to slow growth in the non-Medicare, non-Medicaid sectors of the health system, in turn, would exert some downward pressure on growth rates in the public programs. Moreover, CBO assumes that under current law, the federal government would make regulatory changes aimed at slowing spending growth on federal health programs and that Medicare beneficiaries' demand for health care services would decline as Medicare premiums and cost-sharing amounts consumed a growing share of their income. The combined effects of those factors would be to reduce Medicare's excess cost growth by one-fourth of the reduction for all other nonfederal health care spending.

e. CBO's baseline assumes that the sustainable growth rate (SGR) mechanism will reduce Medicare's physician payment rates by about 5 percent annually through 2016. CBO's alternative scenario assumes that Congress will prevent these reductions as it has since 2003 and will instead tie payment rates to the Medicare economic index, which measures inflation in the inputs used for physician's services.

f. Based on the assumption that the growth of excess cost for Medicare continues at its average rate from 1975 to 2005, 2.4 percentage points. The historical rates of cost growth remove the effect of growth in the number of beneficiaries and the effect of changes in the age composition of the population.

Table 3-5. *How to Offset an Increase in Medicare Spending of 1 Percent of GDP by 2030*

| Factor | Policy change |
|---|---|
| Age of eligibility | Increase from age 65 to age 69. |
| Scope of benefits | Decrease proportion of cost covered by Medicare by one-sixth. |
| Premiums | Increase 125 percent over currently scheduled levels. |
| Discretionary government spending | Cut by 14 percent.[a] |
| Payroll tax | Raise from 2.9 percent to 5.1 percent. |
| Income tax surcharge | Boost all marginal income tax rates from 10, 15, 25, 28, 33, 35 percent to 11, 17, 30, 35, 37, and 40 percent, respectively.[b] |
| New tax | Introduce broadly based value added tax at a rate of 2 percent.[c] |

a. Assumes that 2030 discretionary spending would remain the same in relation to GDP as it was in 2006.

b. Assumes that increased tax rates do not have any effect on the tax base.

c. Based on estimate in CBO, *Reducing the Deficit: Spending and Revenue Options* (March 1997). CBO stopped presenting estimates of added revenue from tax options after this report because the emergence of projected budget surpluses obviated the need for revenue increases. It has not resumed publishing estimates of revenues from a value added tax since then.

The case for increasing the Medicare eligibility age is weak on any grounds other than simple cost cutting. Currently, more than two-thirds of workers claim Social Security before age sixty-five and more than 90 percent before age seventy.[57] If those aged sixty-five to sixty-nine were allowed to buy into Medicare at an actuarially fair price, many would find the price unaffordable and become uninsured. A subsidy sufficient to prevent the loss of coverage would erode most of the savings.[58] Embedding an increase in the Medicare eligibility age in a comprehensive and effective program to encourage workers to retire later than they now do might make sense, but simply raising Medicare's age of eligibility would abandon one fundamental purpose of the program—to ensure that the elderly have access to health care. In addition, raising the age of eligibility would cause some workers to defer retirement in order to retain coverage at their place of work. These workers would raise average premiums for employers. Employers would have increased incentives either to drop sponsorship of health insurance plans or to boost the share of costs borne directly by workers, which would cause some workers of all ages to opt out of coverage.

REDUCE COVERAGE. Reducing Meicare's share of spending on beneficiaries' health care by one-sixth would lower overall Medicare spending by
1 percent of GDP. Such a decrease could be achieved by raising deductibles
or cost sharing. It could also be achieved by curtailing certain benefits, such
as the number of covered hospital days.

Most beneficiaries now regard Medicare coverage as inadequate, as indicated by their interest in supplemental coverage. Scaling back coverage
would likely shift financial burdens to other payers, including Medicaid and
beneficiaries themselves. The cost to the health care system of uncompensated care would rise, as would the demand for special hospital payments
to offset such costs.

INCREASE PREMIUMS. Without further legislative change, Medicare premiums are projected to grow for three reasons. Part B premiums will
increase because Part B outlays are projected to outpace income growth.
Part D premiums for drug benefits are also expected to grow faster than
income. And Congress in 2003 enacted gradual increases in Part B premiums for upper-income beneficiaries. To generate an additional 1 percent of
GDP, overall premiums would have to more than double by 2030. This
increase might well include premiums for Part A as well as increased premiums for Parts B and D. In each case, premiums could be tied to income,
although income-related premiums alone would be insufficient given the
large proportion of seniors with low income.[59]

Raising premiums except for seniors with relatively high incomes would
be problematic. Out-of-pocket spending on health care is projected to
claim three-fifths of seniors' Social Security checks by 2030 and over 80
percent by midcentury. Further premium increases would exacerbate this
problem.[60]

REDUCE OTHER BUDGET OUTLAYS. Congress might elect to offset
increases in Medicare spending with cuts in other government outlays.
According to projections of the Congressional Budget Office, total government spending, apart from health care and interest on the public debt,
will absorb approximately 14 percent of GDP in 2030.[61] This total includes
such long-term mandatory commitments as Social Security and such high-
priority discretionary outlays as national defense. Still, all government outlays are subject to change over the next quarter century. It would take a 14
percent cut in discretionary federal government spending to offset
Medicare's financing gap by 1 percent of GDP in 2030.

RAISE PAYROLL TAXES. Most Part A Medicare spending is offset by a dedicated payroll tax. The current Medicare payroll tax yields 1.4 percent of

GDP. To increase revenue by 1 percent of GDP by 2030, the payroll tax rate would have to be raised from 2.9 percent to 5.1 percent of total earnings.

RAISE INCOME TAXES AND EARMARK THEM TO MEDICARE. In 2007 total revenues from the personal income tax equaled 8.6 percent of GDP. That yield could be increased by taxing currently exempt income, curtailing deductions, or raising rates. Increased rates would lower reported income by encouraging avoidance and evasion. If one ignores base erosion, the rate increases listed in table 3-5 would boost revenue by 1 percent of GDP by 2030. Skewing increases to those with high incomes would be progressive but would also hit workers who already pay 1.45 percent of all their earnings to the program.

INTRODUCE A NEW VALUE ADDED TAX. Among developed nations, the United States alone does not impose a national value added tax (VAT). The base of typical VATs, like that of the retail sales tax (RST), is personal consumption. Most states and some localities now impose RSTs. These taxes could be integrated and administered jointly with a national VAT. Value added tax bases can allow many exclusions or only a few. A VAT with a relatively broad base would apply to about three-quarters of all consumption. Imposed on such a base, a 2 percent rate would yield approximately 1 percent of GDP by 2030.

All policies listed in table 3-5 would be controversial. None may be desirable. But some will likely be necessary to avoid a large fiscal gap. To maintain Medicare benefits promised under current law will be difficult. To expand services will be an even larger challenge. Nor will Medicare be the only source of fiscal pressure. Medicaid and other publicly supported health care outlays will also be rising. Simultaneously, the same pressures will be pushing up private health care spending. Thus the Medicare reform debate will inevitably become a test of national priorities.

## Overview of Alternatives

A debate on how to restructure Medicare and close the gap between projected spending and revenues is long overdue. It will undoubtedly revolve around two key issues. First, projected increases in health care spending will put enormous pressure on the federal budget. Second, Medicare is not currently structured to provide the best-health-care-for-the-buck to its beneficiaries. Most of the remainder of this book describes and evaluates three broad approaches to its structural reform.

The first would simplify the system but retain its social insurance structure, on the assumption that the use of government taxing authority to pay for a single set of benefits for all eligible beneficiaries offers the most promising and least costly way to provide health care to the elderly and people with disabilities. The goal would be to rationalize coverage; to use payment policy, research, and information technology to direct patients to cost-effective medical interventions; and to eliminate the complexity resulting from dividing Medicare into separate parts, each with its own rules and administrative framework. Chapter 4 explains how this approach would work.

The second approach, premium support, would replace the current system with a capped, per person payment that beneficiaries would use to buy health insurance. The government would define standards for qualifying insurance. Enrollees could buy insurance that costs more or less than the payment they receive. They would pay any additional cost themselves and keep any savings. The emphasis would be on market competition among insurers to hold down costs and force changes in the delivery system. This approach has been put forth in various forms by policy analysts and elected officials, most recently in the design of the drug benefit. Chapter 5 lays out this reform strategy.

The third strategy would make individuals responsible for paying expenses up to a relatively high deductible. Beneficiaries would have access to tax-favored, government-subsidized savings accounts from which medical expenses could be paid. Funds in these accounts not used for health care could be used for other purposes with a small penalty. The government would also give beneficiaries a voucher they could use to buy insurance that would cover most outlays in excess of the deductible. The key idea is that if people are spending "their own money" for an increased share of health care spending, they will exercise greater care in selecting providers and bargain more aggressively, thereby policing quality and price more effectively than they do now. This approach to Medicare and to health care financing in general has been advocated by the administration of President George W. Bush. It is the subject of chapter 6.

Elements of each approach may well be combined in any politically acceptable proposal. However, we assess each approach to Medicare reform in its pure form for its ability to promote access, improve quality, and contain costs, goals that are mutually inconsistent, at least in part. Controlling costs by squeezing physician compensation would reduce access by discouraging physicians from seeing Medicare patients. Extending benefits or lowering cost sharing would improve access but raise program costs. Enabling a poorly performing solo doctor in a rural community to continue practicing increases physical access to care but sacrifices the technically better care that patients would receive if they were referred to distant multispecialty medical centers. As chapter 7 makes clear, Medicare reform will entail tradeoffs among Medicare's goals, the strategies proposed to achieve them, and the politics of reform. In the end, however, continuing to ensure that the elderly and people with disabilities receive coverage approximating that enjoyed by the rest of the population will require additional revenue.

# 4 | Strengthening Medicare as a Social Insurance Program

Medicare was originally designed as—and for the most part remains—a *social insurance* program. Social insurance provides collective protection against certain risks such as involuntary unemployment or loss of income because of retirement, disability, or death of a breadwinner.[1] Under Medicare, this protection consists of uniform coverage of the costs of participants' health care regardless of their income or wealth and is financed largely from broadly based taxes. Medicare's uniform benefit structure simplifies administration and avoids the stigma commonly associated with programs targeted to the poor.[2] Because this insurance is either free (Part A) or heavily subsidized (Part B), take-up is virtually universal. And because of its inclusive nature, the program draws widespread political support, which has insulated the program from severe budget cuts. However, Medicare has not adapted quickly to changing health needs and best practices. Coverage has remained fragmentary. Payment policies, until recently, have done almost nothing to discourage low-benefit care or to promote high-quality care.

One strategy for reforming Medicare would deal with these problems while retaining the program's traditional social insurance character—keeping it a predominantly tax-financed program that pays directly for medical services without regard for beneficiary income or wealth. However, numerous other changes would be made. Benefits would be updated and rationalized. The rules governing deductibles and cost sharing would be simplified. A cap on total spending by beneficiaries would be added to preclude catastrophic financial loss. Program administration would be redesigned to increase attention to the quality of health care.[3] In accordance with the tradition of social insurance, this proposal would not use risk-based, private insurers to pay for any Medicare-covered services—although private companies would continue to be employed to help administer the program.[4] Insurers could help organize delivery systems—such as diabetes management programs—but would not assume full financial risk for any population group or any class of benefits.

As a social insurance program, Medicare rests on the rationale that affordable access to care is best achieved through public administration, pooled purchasing, and policies designed to serve the entire Medicare population. This rationale, and its evolution in the United States, has important implications for any efforts to improve Medicare's access, quality, and cost control.

## Origins

Social insurance originated in Bismarckian Germany of the late 1800s in the form of pensions designed to protect workers and their families from some of the economic risks of the Industrial Revolution. The concept eventually spread to health care. Over the course of the twentieth century, it was adopted throughout the world's developed countries. In the United States, pressure for social insurance began mounting in the 1910s, abetted by the Progressive movement's call for government programs to protect workers against financial risks from accident or illness. The Great Depression led to the enactment of Social Security in 1935, which became the model for Medicare, created three decades later.

Like Social Security, Medicare rests on the belief that benefits for seniors and other groups should be available universally, that the federal government should administer them, and that they should be mostly tax financed. The rationale for this approach is that some risks are better managed collectively than individually or through markets.[5] Its roots are variously said to lie in altruism, egalitarianism, or even Judeo-Christian principles.[6] President Lyndon Johnson invoked the Bible at the Medicare signing ceremony: "And this is not just our tradition—or the tradition of the Democratic Party—or even the tradition of the Nation. It is as old as the day it was first commanded: 'Thou shalt open thine hand wide unto thy brother, to thy poor, to thy needy, in thy land.'"[7]

Some believe that health care should be available as a simple right and thus should not be distributed through markets. They see health as a component of the "common good" essential to productivity, equal opportunity, and social equilibrium.[8] According to Arnold Relman, former editor of the *New England Journal of Medicine,* a social and moral compact exists between patients and doctors that should preclude profit-seeking insurers, hospitals, and physician groups from the delivery of health care.[9] Health insurers in particular have come under scrutiny for allegedly avoiding enrolling and paying bills for sick people and diverting resources from patient care to marketing and profits.[10] Health insurers' profit margins are low in comparison with those of other industries but have increased rapidly as health expenditures have risen.[11] While social insurance need not remove either the profit motive from the provision of health care or participation by private insurers, it does limit and regulate their roles.

The two largest U.S. social insurance programs—Social Security and Medicare—originated under Democratic administrations. Both were enacted over Republican opposition. As those programs gained popularity, partisan disagreement waned—until the mid-1990s, when the ideological divide over social insurance reemerged.[12] In 1995, as part of the Republican revolution, Speaker of the House of Representatives Newt Gingrich (R-Ga.) expressed the hope that Medicare would "wither on the vine," to be replaced by competing private insurance plans. Although trust in government was low during this period, trust in such private health care institutions as health maintenance organizations and insurance companies was even lower. Gingrich's wish remained unfulfilled.

In 2003, however, two new measures, enacted with strong Republican support, redirected the program away from traditional social insurance principles. First, the new Medicare drug benefit provided for a risk-adjusted, flat dollar payment—a "defined contribution"—for prescription drug insurance, administered entirely by competing private insurance plans. Within bounds, each plan sets its own premium, cost sharing, list of covered drugs (or formulary), and pharmacy network. Coverage therefore varies from person to person and place to place. The law prohibits the government from negotiating prices for prescription drugs. The government does not guarantee drug coverage but rather subsidizes private coverage. Traditional Medicare, in contrast, ensures access to specific services—or a "defined benefit."

The second step was to revamp the private plan component of Medicare and rename it "Medicare Advantage." The law increased flexibility and funding for private plans, leading more to participate. It also authorized a demonstration under which Medicare's payments for fee-for-service enrollees would be capped beginning in 2010 to allow for "fair competition" between the social insurance and private insurance plans. As a consequence, Medicare policy has in recent years shifted away from social insurance in law—and increasingly in enrollment.[13]

Because of such periodic political shifts, the debate over whether Medicare should remain a traditional social insurance program or be converted into a premium support or a consumer-directed program will continue. As soon as the Democrats regained congressional majorities in 2007, they initiated debates on whether the Medicare Modernization Act's bar on government negotiation of drug prices should be sustained. Other proposals soon emerged to reduce payments to private plans in Medicare. As the chair of the House Ways and Means Subcommittee on Health stated, "Requiring the Secretary to negotiate for lower drug prices is just one small step in the fight against Medicare privatization and the conservative push to end the Medicare entitlement."[14]

## How an Improved Social Insurance Medicare Would Work

A reformed Medicare that preserves its social insurance structure would build on the current system and address its weaknesses. It would continue to pay health care providers directly. The way that beneficiaries enroll and receive benefits would not change. Instead the reforms would focus on correcting the various shortcomings outlined in chapter 3: weak or nonexistent quality incentives, the need to align coverage policy with what works and what is valuable, benefit gaps (which cause most beneficiaries to seek secondary insurance), and blunt payment rates that bear little relationship to cost or value. These problems are not inherent in social insurance but specific to Medicare. Other nations operate social insurance programs that have resolved them in whole or in part, as have other insurers in the United States.

Medicare's performance could be improved in several major ways. Guidelines for use and cost sharing could be structured to encourage patients to use cost-effective medical care. Medicare could be empowered to invest in research to improve quality and lower cost. Finally, Medicare's governance could be modified to increase flexibility and minimize political manipulation in setting program rules. To simplify the program, Parts A and B would be merged. To reaffirm Medicare as social insurance, Part C would be eliminated, and the Part D drug benefit would be folded into the core program. These changes could have a large impact on cost, access, and quality.

## Benefit Reform

Under the social insurance concept, Medicare would return to one menu of covered benefits, deductibles, and cost sharing for all beneficiaries. The rationale for a single set of defined benefits is that the gains—uniform protections, low administrative costs, and leverage on providers to hold down fees—would outweigh the costs of not gratifying differences in insurance tastes.

The process for changing Medicare coverage would be overhauled. Currently, Congress determines the major service categories, their amount, duration, and scope, and their associated cost sharing. It delegates to the executive branch the power to determine coverage of specific therapies. Both branches are subject to political pressures. For example, Congress has added coverage and reduced cost sharing for breast cancer more than for other forms of cancer that have weaker political support. Congress selectively added preventive services recommended by the U.S. Preventive Services Task Force, but it also included a "Welcome to Medicare" electrocardiogram in 2003, which is not medically indicated. Politics influences executive as well as legislative decisions. After intense lobbying from a member of Congress and an industry, Medicare approved coverage of certain costly PET scans for Alzheimer's in 2004, despite the absence of evidence that the procedure affects therapy or outcomes.[15] Medicare's decisions on coverage and cost sharing should be based on clinical merit and cost-effectiveness. To pursue these ends, a new entity within Medicare would determine coverage of major benefit categories. Medicare would enjoy administrative independence from other executive-level agencies, and senior mangers would be appointed for staggered terms and be removable only for cause. These reforms would have little immediate effect on Medicare's benefit coverage or program costs as they would be implemented over time.

A SCIENCE-BASED BENEFITS POLICY. To move toward evidence-based benefit design, Congress would give Medicare increased authority over coverage. Medicare could add or subtract benefits, modify cost sharing, and adjust benefit limits in amount, duration, and scope as long as such changes follow a science-based and accountable process that does not significantly change program costs. To ensure rigor and transparency in its decision-making, Medicare would need to expand its use of experts through coverage advisory panels. Such panels are already in use, but only for narrow decisions. The recommendations of these panels would form the basis of a new, annual report that would recommend coverage policy for the following year. Because such a policy would allow major changes in the program, some external group, such as the Medicare Payment Advisory Commission (MedPAC), would review these decisions. If such changes significantly raised expenditures, Congress would have to approve them before they took effect. Thus Congress would retain political control over decisions that materially change spending but would adopt rules that would strengthen the power of expert panels relying on scientific evidence to design benefits.

Other countries and other U.S. programs base coverage policy on science to a greater extent than does Medicare. For example, Britain's National Health Service uses the results of studies of the cost and clinical implications of various new medical technologies carried out by the National Institute for Health and Clinical Excellence in setting coverage policies.[16] Australia formulates drug coverage policy entirely on evidence reviews. The U.S. Agency for Healthcare Research and Quality and some states have begun to fund comparative effectiveness research and evidence-based practice centers. Proposals also exist to expand comparative effectiveness research in the United States. One survey found that 40 percent of health plans used formal cost-effectiveness analysis in determining coverage policy.[17] Virtually all insurers have "pharmacy and therapeutic" committees to inform decisions about what to include in drug formularies. And MedPAC has recommended that Medicare make greater use of clinical and cost-effectiveness research in its policy setting. Given its size, Medicare has much greater capacity to develop such information and much more to gain from doing so than would any private entity.[18]

Some simple examples illustrate the importance of such information. Research indicates that overall health care spending is minimized if some drugs are provided free to patients or if patients are paid to take them. The resulting savings in reduced hospitalization and use of physician services more than pays for the added drug costs.[19] To encourage use of services that have large clinical and economic value, such as hypertension screening, Medicare could decide to pay fully for the services, with no co-payment. For services of little value or for which better and cheaper alternatives are available, Medicare might pay providers little or impose high cost sharing on patients. Variations in cost sharing have been shown to shape beneficiaries' use of care.[20] Such information is particularly important for designing drug coverage, which would become Medicare's responsibility under the social insurance model.

Because reliable evidence on the effectiveness of most services is not yet available, these techniques would be applied gradually, as information accumulates. Considerable time and a large research investment would be needed to implement such a system. So would procedures to resolve disputes, given the complexity and sensitivity of decisions affecting human health. Physicians would retain the authority to use services that Medicare did not rank as most cost-effective. If a large fraction of physicians overrode a particular policy, Medicare would be obliged to consider whether the policy should be changed. But individual providers who consistently overrode Medicare coverage policy would come under an extra degree of review.

PREMIUMS AND SUPPLEMENTAL COVERAGE. A core principle of social insurance is that benefits should be available on the same terms to all enrollees. This principle implies uniform premiums and cost sharing for everyone. Medicare does not consistently follow this principle. All beneficiaries except those with low-incomes eligible for premium assistance paid the same Part B premium until 2007. Since then, Part B premiums have been income-related for upper-income enrollees. In addition, those beneficiaries who choose to receive Medicare coverage through Part C may pay more or less than enrollees in the traditional program do, depending on whether the plans' bids are high or low and whether they offer extra benefits or reduced charges. Similarly, each prescription drug plan sets its own premium for drug coverage under Part D.

Making Medicare a pure social insurance model implies the elimination of Parts C and D as well as the income-related premium. To prevent this consolidation from increasing budget outlays, the program would change the structure of premiums. The Part B premium would become a programwide charge, the amount of which would approximately offset the same percentage of costs that the current, varied premiums do today. With the disappearance of revenue from the income-related premium, the original Part B premium would go up by about 3 percent.[21] How a standard drug benefit premium affects beneficiaries would depend both on what they pay now and how well the new system constrains spending.

Beyond the premium for basic coverage, Medicare would offer an option for supplemental coverage. This option would narrow the benefit gaps that cause most Medicare enrollees to seek a second—and sometimes a third—insurance policy. Multiple insurance generates additional admin-

istrative and selling costs and thus tends to be uneconomical and ineffi-
cient. Medicare-operated supplemental insurance could take several forms.
One proposal, called Medicare Extra, would have a single deductible of
$250, with coinsurance for all Medicare-covered services set at 10 percent
(25 percent for prescription drugs), and an annual limit of $3,000 (in
2004 dollars) on out-of-pocket spending. Assuming there is no government subsidy, a monthly premium of $95 for this extra protection would
have been sufficient in 2004 to pay for the reduced cost sharing, enhanced
services, administrative costs, and induced increase in service use.[22] Other
proposals for Medicare-run supplemental coverage would offer a choice of
how much to reduce cost sharing—say, to either 5 or 10 percent.[23] The
same evidence-based process used to determine benefits for the core program could be applied in setting supplemental benefits. Beneficiaries who
decided to buy enhanced coverage would have the supplemental premium
added to the base Medicare premium.

Whatever its specific design, the premium would be calibrated on the
assumption that all who are eligible will take the added coverage. To minimize adverse selection—that is, to reduce the tendency for those with
higher-than-average demand for care to enroll selectively—the program
would require beneficiaries who forgo enhanced coverage when they join
Medicare to pay an extra charge if they decide to buy it later on.[24] Employers who offer retiree health coverage and states that run Medicaid would be
encouraged to buy enhanced coverage for Medicare-eligible beneficiaries.
The premium would be the same for all participants.

Private Medigap insurance would not be prohibited but would probably
not be viable. The new supplemental option would have lower overhead
costs than any private plan as well as the imprimatur of Medicare. In addition to giving purchasers added coverage, an integrated supplemental insurance option would enhance Medicare's capacity to manage costs and use.
Currently, supplemental insurers have no incentive to invest in services
that reduce the use or improve the quality of services they do not cover.
Enhanced Medicare would facilitate policies that hold out these promises,
such as comprehensive care coordination.

In accordance with the principles of social insurance, premiums for
Medicare or its new supplemental coverage would not vary by location.
However, costs of delivering uniform benefit packages differ widely from
place to place because prices and use of those services vary. Accordingly,
beneficiaries and providers in low-cost areas and their elected representatives
would have legitimate reason to believe that uniform premiums and cost-

sharing rates will force them to subsidize beneficiaries in areas with high Medicare outlays who have had similar incomes and paid similar taxes. It is not known, however, to what extent these cost variations reflect differences in age, disease incidence, service prices, or use of health care services (and the extent to which any difference in use goes for medically beneficial services). Hence it is not clear whether variable premiums would be fair or medically efficient.

### Payment Reform

The current Medicare fee-for-service system has come under criticism on several fronts. Most providers consider its rates inadequate, but then many of them feel the same way about private payment rates. Even if they are disgruntled, Medicare's market position is so dominant that they can afford to refuse patients only if reimbursement is grossly inadequate, and sometimes not even then. Not only is Medicare the primary payer for many services, but private insurers frequently use its rates as a benchmark for their own. Unlike private insurers, however, Medicare has been slow to modify and update its reimbursement systems, in part because Congress must enact the changes.

Perhaps the most serious criticism of Medicare's payment policy is that it is based on the cost of providing a service without regard for the benefits that service generates. As a result, Medicare pays more for complex and resource-intensive care, even if it is ineffective, than it pays for simple, inexpensive, highly beneficial services. In treating heart attacks, for example, handsome payments encourage high-tech coronary artery bypass surgery and angioplasty that are life-saving for some patients but of marginal value for many. At the same time, Medicare pays little or nothing for prescribing and encouraging the use of beta-blockers and aspirin, which are cheap, effective, and medically indicated for almost everyone. Such incentives contribute to the finding that, in the case of heart attacks, areas with higher-than-average per patient costs produce worse-than-average survival rates.[25]

This problem could be ameliorated if Medicare had broader authority to modify payment policies. Medicare administrators could be empowered to change payment policies without congressional approval if approved by MedPAC or other experts, and if the impact on cost was below legislated thresholds. Some of this authority already exists; for instance, the Centers for Medicare and Medicaid Services (CMS) has extensive rule-making authority. Congress could retain the authority to override delegated decisions but might adopt voting rules to discourage itself from second-guessing—for example, it could impose a Senate rule requiring a sixty-vote super-majority to override such changes.

Medicare could use such authority to establish explicit rewards for improvements in quality. The Institute of Medicine (IOM) and other health policy leaders have already called for "fundamental changes in approaches to health care payment" to improve quality.[26] The IOM recommends financial rewards for quality performance. When the United Kingdom began increasing the income of primary care physicians if they met a number of quality benchmarks, follow-up studies confirmed that these incentives were working.[27] Medicare is in a better position than any private payer to implement such reforms because it has accumulated data on over 40 million enrollees and accounts for a large share of the income of hospitals and physicians. With its powerful data systems, it could monitor indicators of quality based both on adherence to best procedures and on medical outcomes as well as payment patterns to design payment systems that align reimbursement with value.

Medicare should also be allowed to test and adopt innovative payment mechanisms. Its current demonstration authority is strong, but successful ideas often languish because of congressional inaction.[28] Medicare could, with MedPAC approval, adopt alternative payment systems. It should have authority to seek bids for the treatment of specific medical conditions such as diabetes or other chronic diseases. Demonstrations would be used to show how social insurance can, in some areas, use market competition both to lower prices and to encourage innovation. Perhaps most important, the program should identify and assess cost-effective methods of caring for patients with multiple illnesses, as such patients account for most of Medicare's spending. In short, Medicare could continually test, evaluate, implement, modify, and, if necessary, overhaul its payment policies.

If prescription drugs are covered by Medicare rather than by separate, privately administered insurance plans, it will be necessary to decide how to pay manufacturers for prescription drugs and how much to charge patients. Several possibilities exist. One would be to replace the private, risk-based prescription drug plans with multiple, non-risk-based pharmaceutical benefit managers (PBMs). Since both the premium and benefit design would be standardized, such plans could compete for enrollees on the basis of price, quality of service, and drug management only. Or Medicare could contract with one PBM per region to administer the benefit, much as it now contracts with private companies to administer Parts A and B. The PBM would be selected through periodic open competition based on price discounts and quality, similar to the approach taken by most large employers.[29] Alternatively, Medicare could negotiate drug prices directly with drug manufacturers. This approach is used by other government programs, such as the Veterans Health Administration, and by other nations.

These options might also be combined in some fashion. For example, Medicare could negotiate the prices of new or one-of-a-class drugs, while PBMs negotiate and compete for lower prices for drugs with equivalent substitutes.[30] If Medicare were to act as the sole negotiator for all drugs, drug development would suffer because the bargaining power of a single monopsonistic purchaser would threaten profits and undermine financial backing for drug research. Basing drug prices on their comparative clinical and cost-effectiveness, however, could enhance incentives for drug companies to deliver high-value rather than "me-too" drugs. Whatever the specific approach, determination of prices for drugs under a social insurance model would not be delegated to private insurers but would be made by Medicare or by PBMs acting for Medicare.

As for pricing drugs to patients, private plans frequently charge patients flat dollar co-payments in two or more "tiers." Low-tier co-payments are applied to "preferred" drugs: generics, high-value drugs within a therapeutic class, and drugs for which there are no substitutes. Higher-tier co-payments are charged for other drugs. To secure discounts from manufacturers, PBMs often promise to classify a drug as "preferred." Tiered co-payments not only shape patients' decisions about what drugs to use, but also protect them from most of the very large differences in price between patented drugs and generics.

Medicare could instead use "reference pricing," a method employed in Germany, Norway, the Netherlands, New Zealand, and Canada. Under reference pricing, Medicare would define classes of drugs and pay a flat sum for all drugs within the class. Usually the reference payment is set at the price of the least costly drug in the class or an average of relatively low-cost drugs. The beneficiary must pay all of the cost above the reference amount, encouraging price competition among drug substitutes. Reference pricing, like tiered co-payments, faces technical difficulties. One tricky but very important question is how to determine which drugs belong in the same class. Another is how to allay the strong political resistance to setting a Medicare formulary.[31] Still another is how to set the reference dosage and package size (prices routinely differ on the basis of package size and pill strength). It is also necessary to decide where in the distribution of possible prices the reference price should be set.[32]

These methods of setting prices differ in their impact on patients and on drug companies. Tiered co-payments shield patients from most of the difference between the cost of patented drugs and generics, whereas reference pricing exposes patients to all of the difference. Accordingly, reference pricing tends to hold down the prices that drug companies can charge for patented drugs for which there is a sufficiently close therapeutic substitute. Advocates of reference pricing see this effect as a virtue because it means consumers save money. Critics consider it a flaw because low prices reduce incentives to develop new drugs. Under either approach, Medicare would simplify the cost-sharing system for its drug benefit by having a uniform deductible and applying cost sharing nationwide.

### Quality Systems

Medicare was established to pay for health care, not to manage it. Founding legislation barred it from influencing the practice of medicine. Medicare is required to pay any licensed provider who renders care to beneficiaries and follows program rules and regulations, regardless of the quality of that care. For these reasons, the program has done little to ensure that indicated care is offered, to discourage inappropriate care, or to promote efficiency. This neglect of quality has not been confined to Medicare. Beyond licensing, public policy has paid limited attention to the quality of care actually rendered, patient safety, and systemwide reforms to improve quality. The notable exception is that, in instances of demonstrable negligence, patients may sue for malpractice.

Goaded by analyses documenting the prevalence of avoidable medical errors, hospital administrators, physicians, and employers have launched efforts to improve the quality of care.[33] Medicare has joined this movement—collecting data on quality and testing "pay for performance" to link financial rewards with good performance. To date, however, the enormous power of the nation's largest health care payer to improve health care quality for its beneficiaries—and, indirectly, for the nation—has barely been tapped. A revitalized social insurance program has the potential to align benefit design and payment policy to elicit high-quality, value-oriented care.

If this reform strategy were adopted, Medicare would use its purchasing power as a major payer to set minimum performance standards and targets for optimal performance, and generally to "raise the bar" on quality. These efforts could take many forms. We list three.

First, Medicare could use the leverage of professional norms to improve health care quality. Historically, licensed providers have by and large been self-regulated. They have policed their own errors, often in closed-door medical reviews. Regulators were reluctant to use blunt enforcement tools, such as the revocation of hospital privileges and licenses, but the increasing frequency of medical malpractice litigation and recent research into patient safety have opened the process. Moreover, since health care professionals remain acutely sensitive to the norms of their own medical communities, those standards can greatly abet reform. The Veterans Health Administration, once scorned for the poor quality of its health care, transformed itself into one of the nation's most highly regarded medical systems, in part by promoting the use of feedback loops to encourage providers to improve their performance.[34] Several states have developed regional quality forums to improve quality.[35] These forums typically gather data, search for patterns, and feed the results—which include comparisons with local, regional, and national processes and outcomes—back to providers and facilities.

With its current repository of data and capacity to generate more, Medicare could ably sponsor such regional quality forums, as well as support research to identify good and bad practices. Local medical leadership could tailor each forum's work to local problems. Demonstration programs are showing that care coordination and support services are essential to positive outcomes for complicated illnesses. The need for skilled home health services is particularly urgent where nursing homes are scarce or extended families are uncommon. The provision of each of these services depends on local resources. In addition, regional forums may be able to gain the trust of local providers more readily than could national organizations. The forums could communicate information privately as well as publicly, eventually supplying consumers with information on provider performance.[36]

Second, Medicare could play a pivotal role in "raising the bar" on quality through the use of its purchasing power. Medicare already enforces minimum safety standards in health care institutions. To go even further, it could levy penalties on hospitals that do not have systems for preventing disease and the incorrect administration of drugs. It could use its capital payments to persuade hospitals to invest in buildings, equipment, software, and training. Even if Congress is unwilling to modify the "any-willing-provider" rule, Medicare could be authorized to set payment differentials for above-average and below-average performers. It could also be authorized to exclude error-prone providers.

Recent experience in Germany indicates how such incentives might be applied. German hospitals are required to submit data on measures of quality developed in collaboration with outside experts and providers. Poorly performing hospitals are asked to participate in a "structured dialogue" designed to improve performance. Hospitals that do not improve after several rounds of dialogue may lose payments. In practice, all hospitals have improved, and the project has been extended to ambulatory care.[37] The clear lesson here is that a system of measuring quality, reporting the results, providing incentives, and, as a last resort, imposing penalties can encourage providers to adopt practices that promote quality and reduce errors. Medicare is uniquely positioned to administer such quality-improving programs.

Third, Medicare could invest in projects designed to improve quality. Such investments are what economists call public goods—products that should be freely available because, once developed, added use does not deplete the stock available for others. Profit-oriented organizations that serve only part of the population invest less than is socially optimal in such goods because they reap only a fraction of the total benefits. To date, Medicare has made few investments of this kind because it has a tight budget for administration, devoid of unrestricted funds to invest in what could produce long-run gains for the program or for the health care system. If Medicare had investment authority, it could jump-start research on the comparative effectiveness of health services or invest in such tools as information technology. Medicare could lead the nation in developing electronic health records and creating a paperless administrative system. Aggressive implementation and use of health information technology could not only save money—$81 billion a year after fifteen years, according to one study—but could also improve the management of complex cases and facilitate the monitoring of quality.[38] Once developed, such methods would be freely available for use outside Medicare. Although some improvements could be achieved through regulation, front-end investments are also needed.[39] Medicare could devote a fraction of program outlays or a flat sum to such investments.

## Management

Because of Medicare's current structure, its officials have limited ability to manage the program. Its administrator, or chief executive officer, reports to the secretary of the Department of Health and Human Services. The department responds to the White House. Other executive branches have a say in policy as well, notably the Office of Management and Budget and the Department of the Treasury. On the legislative side, Congress aggressively oversees Medicare policy decisions and implementation. These multiple and often competing Medicare policymakers constrain and sometimes distort its management decisions. Medicare's administrator is also responsible for Medicaid and the State Children's Health Insurance Programs, which now serve more people than Medicare does. Medicare's administrator and most of its senior staff are political appointees. No administrator has served more than four years. Furthermore, the program is not permitted to make large or quick changes. In light of its responsibilities, the staff is indeed small.[40]

Before Medicare can become more effective as a social insurance program, its management needs to be strengthened and made more independent. One such avenue of reform would be to move authority for administering the program to an independent agency. The administrator would remain a presidential appointee, subject to congressional approval, but would be appointed for a fixed term, subject to termination only for cause. Medicare would be given authority to make a broad range of key decisions—such as what benefits to cover and how to pay for them—with input from experts such as MedPAC but with authority to implement them unless Congress explicitly disapproved. Its staff would be enlarged and relieved of responsibilities for other health programs and policies. The program would no longer be divided into separate parts—A, B, C, and D—and management would be organized around functions. Ideally, Medicare would be managed less like a government agency and more like Kaiser Permanente.

To be sure, increased flexibility would require close oversight, especially to ensure transparency in management's decisionmaking. Reports to Congress would explain major policy changes, and decisions would be open to public comment. Technical decisions would be supervised by advisory panels. And any move involving sizable changes in expenditures would still require congressional action. Congress would retain the authority to revise or reverse any decision made by Medicare administrators through legislation.

## What a Typical Beneficiary Would Encounter

Beneficiaries would not see much difference between this model and their experience with Medicare today. A typical beneficiary—call her Ms. Brown—who is approaching age sixty-five receives a letter informing her of her impending Medicare coverage. She has the choice of purchasing Medicare supplemental insurance. If she does so, the premium for this extra coverage will be added to the premium for the basic program and the total deducted from her Social Security check. She does not choose a separate drug plan with a different premium because this benefit is now folded into the current program. Nor does she need to find a Medigap or Medicare

Advantage plan if she lacks retiree coverage because the Medicare supplemental option will replace it. If she declines supplemental coverage, she can buy it later, but at a higher premium designed to offset adverse selection and the age-related increase in expected health care spending.

Once enrolled, Ms. Brown shares the cost of covered services identified in a publicly available list. This list is set by Medicare, with input from an expert panel. It changes every year as Medicare reviews data on the clinical value and cost of current and new services. An annual letter informs Ms. Brown of changes in coverage and cost sharing. She receives a toll-free number and an Internet site to obtain additional information regarding prescription drugs and other aspects of the program.

Ms. Brown might find her initial premium higher than she expected, but it will not increase with age. If she is healthy, her out-of-pocket costs will be low. Cost-effective preventive care, such as periodic mammograms and flu shots, are free. Depending on her supplemental coverage, she pays a low and predictable share of the cost of a physician visit for minor ailments. She typically pays less to fill a prescription for a generic drug than for a drug still under patent.

Her costs will increase in proportion to use up to a new annual limit on out-of-pocket spending. This limit will be the same for all beneficiaries and will be automatic rather than based on Mrs. Brown's decisions at age sixty-five. If various treatment options are available, coverage policy could influence treatment decisions. Suppose that Ms. Brown develops lower back pain from a herniated disc with pressure on a nerve that causes weakness in her leg and threatens permanent damage if not relieved. If she opts for back surgery, a costly treatment, she will benefit from a limit on out-of-pocket spending. If she opts for medication, a less costly treatment, her cost sharing will depend on whether the drug recommended by her doctor is also recommended by Medicare. A third option might be physical therapy. If Medicare coverage of physical therapy remains limited because of cost pressures on the program, Ms. Brown will have to pay out of pocket for such services, with no limit on her cost exposure. Variation in cost sharing is inevitable because a single benefit package designed to encourage use of high-value services cannot protect all beneficiaries equally. This feature could make Ms. Brown unhappy if her definition of "high value" is different from Medicare's.

Ms. Brown has access to all health care providers except those who elect not to serve Medicare patients or who fail to meet new minimum quality guidelines. Like all beneficiaries, she receives information on the quality of providers in her area. She pays the same amount regardless of which provider she selects. Under premium support or consumer-directed Medicare, in contrast, she would pay different amounts depending on providers' charges. Under a revised social insurance program, however, providers themselves might receive extra payments for superior performance.

Ms. Brown's Medicare experience will change little as she ages. She decides on supplemental coverage upon entering the program. Medicare determines premiums, cost sharing, and coverage policy for her. Her primary decisions are whether to use services, given their cost sharing, and which doctors to see. Such simplicity might seem rigid if Ms. Brown wants a service that is not covered by Medicare. In that case, she might prefer different coverage. But if Ms. Brown values being able to choose which provider to see, this model may suit her well.

## The Devilish Details

The pure social insurance approach outlined here is intended to improve Medicare's performance on access, quality improvement, and cost control. However, three aspects of the plan are likely to be particularly controversial.

### Elimination of Private Plans

The pure social insurance model would eliminate Medicare Advantage (Part C) and the freestanding drug insurance program (Part D). These steps would be objectionable to many. Most of the one-fifth of Medicare beneficiaries enrolled in a Medicare Advantage plan in 2007 received more benefits for lower premiums than did enrollees in standard Medicare. One reason for those extra benefits is that Medicare pays Part C plans more than the costs it incurs for similar enrollees in the standard program.[41] Any attempt to roll back the extra payments might cause an uproar. In 2007, in anticipation of such a proposal, the managed care industry issued a report predicting that such rollbacks would reduce low-income and minority enrollment in private plans, causing these vulnerable beneficiaries to lose preventive and other needed care.[42] These overpayments, critics countered, were setting Medicare on the path to privatization.[43]

Replacing Part D with a single social insurance plan would fuel debate as well. When the drug benefit was established, Medicare enrollees who subscribed to it had to make complex decisions by comparing formularies, deductibles, other cost sharing, and premiums of different plans. By 2008,

43 percent of Medicare beneficiaries had made those decisions.[44] Although the drug benefit in the expanded social insurance plan would be much simpler than the current one, the switch would be disruptive and would produce both "winners" and "losers." Drug companies would fear that price regulation would soon follow and could be counted on to keep beneficiaries on the alert for any faults in the new system. In sum, fewer changes might be needed to strengthen Medicare as a social insurance program than to implement wholly new models such as premium support or consumer-directed Medicare, but the changes would generate fierce resistance from groups whose interests might be adversely affected.

## Delegation from Congress to the Executive Branch

Under social insurance reform, Congress would have to delegate considerable power to Medicare. Historically, Congress has been willing to delegate politically unpopular or technical decisions (such as those relating to air traffic control) to the executive branch but has been loath to transfer authority over major policy decisions, particularly in matters as politically sensitive and expensive as Medicare. The political response to the recommendation of the Bipartisan Commission on the Future of Medicare in 1999 that the government create a Medicare Board and empower it to make major policy and payment decisions illustrates the point. A Democratic Congress and president opposed the idea because, they said, such a board would not be sufficiently accountable to the public. Even if Congress granted such authority, some observers believe that it would intervene whenever decisions of such a group impinged on the interests of constituents or major economic players.

## Even Good Evidence Is Fallible

The reform would rely far more than the current program does on evidence and expertise in setting benefits, formulating payment policies, and promoting quality. It is hard to argue that health care should *not* rest on a sound, scientific base. However, the conclusions of science are always provisional and subject to modification by future research. They are also generally probabilistic—drug A works better than drug B *most of the time*. And they tend to be complex and subject to interpretation, as in "Surgery is indicated only in patients who are sufficiently fit and whose lesions have not developed beyond a certain stage." Furthermore, new research sometimes finds previous therapeutic regimens to be inferior. Such science may not be strong enough to withstand political pressures and the pleadings of those whose interests have been damaged by Medicare's decisions. For many enrollees, decisions in which the costs of a procedure override its positive benefits would smack of rationing. This problem would be particularly intense for chronically ill patients because clear guidelines on what works best are often lacking.

The problem of when to end aggressive care for the terminally ill would be even more difficult. Providers can be counted on to argue that their patients are exceptions to whatever rule Medicare advances or that "cookbook medicine" does not work. Some providers will confound venality with virtue, masking financial self-interest with criticisms of the science that lies behind restrictions on coverage. All the same, the volume and reliability of medical evidence would grow and improve if the largest payer for health care in the country used scientific data in setting benefits and monitoring quality. Medicare would become a more discriminating purchaser of health care than it is now. But even the best science will not resolve all uncertainty; indeed, this uncertainty will pose a practical as well as a political challenge to a system that bases coverage on research findings. As a result, decisions not to cover certain services, or to require large cost sharing for them, would anger some providers. Although physicians and other experts would have a greater role in making Medicare policy decisions, they might still feel financially and professionally threatened by the program's added powers.

## Assessment

Whether one sees these modifications to Medicare as desirable improvements in a system that should retain its character as social insurance or as obstacles to genuine reforms that would move the system away from that model depends on one's larger view of the current program. If today's program is deemed successful but in need of some important but not fundamental fixes, then the proposed changes can be assessed for their marginal effects. If the current system is seen as a structural blunder, then these changes cannot solve its problems. The following assessment takes the first approach, viewing the program as one that meets most of its goals.

### Ensuring Access

The reforms described here preserve a key feature of the current program—in that they give doctors ultimate control over decisions about what services are prescribed. While cost sharing and payment policy would be designed to steer patients and providers toward high-value care, the plan would not require prior authorization for care, nor would it necessitate gatekeepers, staffing limits, or other instruments of cost control that private insurers use to manage care. Access to care, a primary goal of Medicare, would be maintained and might be enhanced by authorizing Medicare to offer supplemental insurance. Currently, Medigap insurance is costly and the availability of some plans is spotty. This option would give all beneficiaries access to a complete menu of supplemental coverage options at a predictable premium. The social insurance model would not use selective provider networks to drive down prices, a threat to access in rural and other underserved areas, where the exclusion of a particular provider may leave people with few good options for care.

### Promoting Quality and Satisfaction

Through its single risk pool, Medicare has already amassed much of the performance data and many of the payment tools required to promote high-quality, cost-effective health care. To date, however, it has made only limited use of these tools. Medicare's very size poses political obstacles to such use. Providers fear that linking quality metrics to payment will reduce their professional autonomy.[45] Also, the science of quality measurement remains imperfect. These obstacles to quality promotion will not be easy to overcome even in a reformed social insurance system.

Regional forums provide the best hope of making this approach workable. The forums would engage local medical leadership, which would act as a source of guidance in place of a distant bureaucracy. Whether this approach would reduce the regional variation in practice patterns that increase service costs without increasing quality is unclear. Perhaps the most promising way for Medicare to boost overall quality would be to establish minimum performance standards. Medicare has demonstrated that it can induce system-wide provision of language services and enforce emergency-room access policy. It could use similar leverage to lift the performance of health providers, to the benefit of Medicare enrollees and the population at large.

Satisfaction with care, another dimension of quality, would likely increase under these reforms. An option for supplemental coverage would likely raise Medicare's already high level of popularity, especially for beneficiaries who value the right to choose providers. However, choice among benefit packages and health plans would vanish. Uniformity would become a serious drawback if benefits failed to keep pace with either science or expectations. Limits on benefits and increased cost sharing, even if backed by scientific evidence, might well reduce satisfaction.

### Controlling Costs

Current projections indicate a bleak financial future for Medicare. Can the reforms we have described contain costs? The answer is that these reforms may slow the growth of spending, but neither these reforms nor those set forth in the next two chapters are sufficient to reduce the need for higher revenue or other painful measures described in chapter 3.

Under the social insurance approach, Medicare would use effectiveness research and cost data to update, modify, and replace payment systems by increasing flexibility. Congress would grant Medicare the power to make such decisions without prior approval, but would retain the authority to review and change Medicare's actions. It would also base coverage policy and cost sharing on scientific evidence and thereby steer patients and providers toward appropriate and efficient care. Not all health services offer the same value. Some have little benefit per dollar spent. Whether systematic application of scientific evidence to coverage policy and cost sharing would hold down spending cannot be known in advance. Cost sharing would remain limited. Out-of-pocket spending would be capped. And physicians might find ways to override any limitations. Furthermore, cost-effective care is not always cheap, and research has shown widespread underuse of indicated therapies.[46]

Neither coverage nor quality policies can wholly offset one central limitation of the fee-for-service payment system, which is also a defining characteristic of traditional Medicare: health care providers prescribe the treatment for the problem they diagnose. They gain financially even if treatments are unneeded or of little benefit. A refined payment policy and institutional oversight of quality can counteract these incentives only to a degree. The proposed changes would improve Medicare's cost control, but whether they would control overall Medicare spending as well as premium support and high-deductible plans is debatable.

## Conclusion

One notable proposal for the reform of Medicare would maintain its social insurance character. Through its single risk pool, the program would directly pay for all covered benefits, including prescription drugs, and would offer integrated supplemental insurance, lessening the need for other supplemental insurance. Its ability to modify how it pays for services would be enhanced. A new policy priority would be to encourage high-quality care through regional forums, mechanisms for excluding poorly performing providers, and research aimed at identifying measures of efficiency and quality.

Social insurance has distinct strengths and weaknesses. It is comparatively simple for enrollees, providers, and taxpayers. For a given premium, payroll tax, and general revenue contribution, the proposed reform would give all people who are elderly or disabled the same benefits. Medicare's success in ensuring access would continue, as would its free choice of doctors and hospitals. The proposal would improve Medicare quality and enable the program to employ prices to guide use. On the other hand, it would offer little choice of insurance coverage. It would rely heavily on prices to control spending and would have few instruments to prevent the overuse of services.

Medicare reform that does not depart from the program's current general structure has one clear advantage over the other major proposals. It has been tried. The benefits of the systems described in chapters 5 and 6 remain by and large speculative. Their transition costs would be high. Whether the well-recognized flaws of social insurance are fatal or fixable is a key question to ask in assessing these options. According to proponents of social insurance, any cure that replaces Medicare with a new arrangement may be worse than the disease.[47] The next two chapters examine those alternatives so that readers can form their own judgments.

# 5 Premium Support

Beginning in the mid-1990s, policy analysts developed and some elected officials endorsed an alternative to traditional Medicare called *premium support*.[1] This term has since been applied to several proposals built around the principle that health care services should be financed by the government but managed by private insurance plans competing on premiums and services. The government would pay for a core set of services. This payment—or "capitation"—would be adjusted on the basis of enrollees' characteristics to reflect differences in expected use of health care. The payment adjustments would reduce insurers' incentives to "cherry-pick"—that is, to seek enrollees with low expected medical use. The Medicare Modernization Act (MMA) adopted this approach for the drug benefit added to Medicare in 2003. Premium support is the principle underlying the Medicare Advantage program. The MMA also authorized a premium support demonstration to begin in 2010.

Proponents of premium support claim that plans will respond to enrollees' preferences more quickly if people can switch plans rather than be forced to remain in one that may or may not respond to pressure for change. Private insurers, unencumbered by government red tape, would be the administrative "hare" to Medicare's bureaucratic "tortoise," introducing innovative administrative procedures and goading providers to adopt cost-reducing and quality-improving therapies. Medicare's use of private plans would extend to retirement years the kind of insurance most people had encountered during their working years. In addition, premium support would give Congress greater capacity to limit spending than traditional Medicare does.

One premium support model suitable for Medicare is similar to what is being used in parts of Medicare Advantage today. Plans would offer an integrated set of benefits with some degree of standardization. Medicare would base its payments to such plans on regional "benchmarks," or averages of plan bids for standard coverage. Plan premiums would be increased or decreased by the difference between the plan bid and the benchmark (if the bid was above the benchmark, the enrollee would pay the difference; if below, the enrollee would receive the difference). This version, one of a variety of possible premium support proposals, is explored in this chapter.

## Origins

Premium support evolved from "managed competition," a term coined by Stanford Business School economist Alain Enthoven.[2] The idea is to control health care spending not by regulating price or imposing explicit coverage limits, but by exposing health care users to the full incremental cost of insurance above a core plan and allowing insurance plans themselves to compete for enrollees by innovating, cutting costs, and improving quality. Heightened price sensitivity on the demand side and intensified competition on the supply side would result, it is claimed, in more care per dollar. At the same time, premium support would mandate certain broad benefit categories and include rules to ensure access to coverage. In addition, government subsidies would be linked to increases in general health costs rather than to an index that is independent of health care. This last feature distinguishes managed competition from voucher plans, which link spending per person to non-health indicators such as income or economic growth. Managed competition was the inspiration for the Health Security Act, President Clinton's failed 1994 health reform plan, which proposed to insure most nonelderly Americans through private plans in regional alliances.[3]

In 1999 premium support graduated from minor-league policy analysis to a major-league policymaking debate when the National Bipartisan Commission on the Future of Medicare laid out a detailed premium support proposal. Although a majority of commission members supported the

proposal, which included other policies such as a low-income drug benefit, it failed to garner the supermajority required under commission rules
to make recommendations to Congress. Several months later, the Clinton
administration put forward a "competitive defined-benefit" model that
had elements of premium support but did not include traditional Medicare
in its capitated payment system. Introduced just before the 2000 elec-
tions, the Democratic-sponsored proposal went nowhere in the
Republican-led Congress.

Four years later, a Republican-controlled White House and Congress
revived managed competition in three parts of the MMA. The newly
enacted drug benefit was to be delivered only through competing private
drug plans paid a flat, per enrollee, risk-adjusted federal fee.[4] If the cost of
providing benefits exceeds this fee, enrollees pay the balance. Private companies, operating under federal rules, compete regionally for enrollees on
the basis of price, benefit design, and service. Competition, it was thought,
would keep drug prices low and satisfaction high. Under a second provision
of the MMA, Medicare Advantage plans—a new name for Part C—were
to be paid in accordance with county or regional "benchmarks." Enrollees'
premiums are based on the difference between that benchmark payment
and the actual plan bid, a structure intended to promote premium competition. In addition, the MMA called for a six-year premium support demonstration to begin in 2010. In an attempt to promote competition, premiums
for Medicare fee-for-service in six metropolitan areas will be set as under
Medicare Advantage, with Medicare's contribution converted to capitation
payments.[5] Although most Medicare beneficiaries have now experienced a
form of premium support through the drug benefit, the impact on costs,
access, quality, and satisfaction of converting all benefits to capitation is not
yet known.

## How Premium Support Would Work

Under premium support, the agency responsible for administering
Medicare would stop setting prices and payment rules for medical
providers, services, and devices and simply subsidize health insurance plans
on behalf of enrollees. Insurers could offer a range of plans, including fee-
for-service insurance similar to traditional Medicare, health maintenance
organizations, and other forms of managed care. Considerable regulation
would be necessary to ensure that premium support operates efficiently
and fairly and provides at least minimum benefits.

## *How Plan Benefits and Cost Sharing Would Be Determined*

Premium support would retain a key element of traditional Medicare: people who contribute payroll taxes during their working years would be guaranteed coverage of core medical services. Though difficult to define, a list of specific core benefits would be established to discourage insurers from trying to use benefits to cherry-pick low-cost enrollees. If wholly unregulated, insurers might offer sports medicine benefits to attract physically active seniors or stint on services for costly illnesses like cancer. Successful cherry-picking is privately profitable but socially wasteful, as costly enrollees will eventually be covered somewhere else in the system.

At the same time, plans would have some flexibility in designing benefits if patients are to be offered more choice of coverage than Medicare now provides. Allowing benefits to vary by plan encourages innovation and choice and enables the market to determine optimal coverage for Medicare's limited financing. The lack of this flexibility in the current program, some argue, is the reason it took Medicare forty years to add coverage of prescription drugs.

A blended policy of mandated and optional benefits could be adopted. Plans would have to offer a standard benefit package with an actuarial value at least equal to that of the current Medicare program. They would have to cover defined services: inpatient hospital services, office visits to physicians, effective preventive services, and critical drugs, for example.[6] Other provisions could also be specified, such as a maximum single deductible and an annual limit on out-of-pocket expenses. In addition, the drug benefit would be folded into the core benefit package. As with current private drug plans in Medicare, formularies and other rules would be subject to review and approval by Medicare. This strategy would require fewer regulatory decisions than are necessary for detailed specification of a benefit package. It also is a way of discovering how to spend a given sum in ways that best promote the health and satisfy the wants of enrollees, assuming that these are insurers' goals. In this way, benefit decisions would be made by private plans to reflect local preferences, but within limits set by Medicare.

Plans could offer benefits beyond the standard package. Unlike the current system, however, premium support would make beneficiaries buy that coverage from the same insurer that delivers the basic benefits. This requirement is essential, because it would internalize in one insurer any demand-increasing effects of supplemental coverage. As with the core benefits, what is offered would be clearly defined and regulated to discourage insurers from using benefits to appeal selectively to low-cost patients. Some standardization also helps markets work by enabling customers to compare the prices and performance of various companies. Hence a critical function of Medicare under premium support would be to provide beneficiaries with information on their plan choices.

### How the Medicare Subsidy Would Be Set

Medicare would stop paying for individual services and instead pay health plans flat sums for providing services to plan enrollees. Government officials would still have to compute payments to plans and adjust them periodically, but eliminating the need for Medicare to set myriad prices would greatly simplify federal administration.

The initial subsidy payment could be set in various ways: at the price of the cheapest plan in an area, at the median or average of the prices of all plans offered in an area, at a national average price, or at locally specific prices based on prevailing practice patterns and service prices. It could be set as "the same dollar amount" or "the same proportion" of the cost of a standard insurance plan. Because local health insurance expenditures vary widely, these alternative subsidy rules would yield quite different results.[7]

Like Medicare Advantage, this version of premium support would base subsidies on "regional benchmarks" computed as the enrollment-weighted average of health plans' bids. The bid is the insurance plan's estimated cost of delivering Medicare's standard benefits in that area for an average beneficiary population. Medicare's subsidy to each plan would be the regional benchmark minus the standard Medicare premium paid by all beneficiaries, adjusted for the risk characteristics of enrollees. Beneficiaries' premiums would approximate what they pay for Medicare under the current system, plus (or minus) the difference between the bids of the plans in which they enroll and the benchmark. If a beneficiary selects a plan that bids less than the benchmark, then that enrollee's premium will be lower than the standard premium by the amount of that difference. If beneficiaries choose plans that bid more than the benchmark, they must pay the full excess in addition to the standard premium. If a plan's bid is higher because it offers supplemental benefits, it will have to report separately the extra premium attributable to extra benefits. This system is designed to encourage plans to keep bids low to attract enrollees and drive out high-bid plans.

Benchmarks would be updated annually to reflect changes in the average expected bid and the previous year's enrollment. Such adjustments would reflect changes in the service menu, service use, and prices. This approach bases the government contribution solely on the competitive bids. Government spending moves up or down with bids. An alternative approach is to keep the growth of Medicare cost in line with that of national spending, namely, by increasing the average subsidy in accordance with the annual growth in national average per capita spending on health care. This rule would maintain the relative generosity of subsidies, which would change with prices and the mix of services nationwide. But it would not reflect any changes in expenditures attributable to the competition set up by premium support.

Both methods for updating Medicare's subsidies distinguish premium support from so-called voucher plans that would tie the government subsidy to some broad economic index, such as the growth in per capita income. Without explicit congressional action, voucher plans would cover progressively smaller shares of health care spending, because those broad indexes have grown more slowly than health care spending.[8] If the Medicare subsidy increase were tied to general price inflation, the erosion would take place even faster, as per capita income typically grows faster than prices. Of course, Congress would be free to raise subsidies to keep pace with health care spending, but the baseline policy has considerable political significance and may be hard to change. Premium support, in contrast, would keep Medicare spending loosely tied to the actual cost of health care for the covered population.

## How to Minimize Risk Selection

Premium support is intended to promote competition in order to achieve efficiency, adaptability, and high quality. It can achieve those outcomes if insurers compete for enrollees by offering good coverage via high-performing providers at a low price—but will be less likely to do so if insurers try to attract healthy beneficiaries and avoid costly ones. Most medical expenditures derive from a small proportion of very costly patients. In 2002 the costliest 5 percent of beneficiaries enrolled in traditional Medicare accounted for 48 percent of total fee-for-service Medicare spending, and the costliest 25 percent accounted for 88 percent.[9] The high concentration of outlays means that the private return to avoiding high-cost enrollees is enormous. In fact, enrollees in Medicare managed care plans have been healthier, younger, and less costly than average. Various policies can reduce the returns to such socially wasteful competition, some of which could be incorporated into premium support.

RISK ADJUSTMENT AND OTHER PAYMENT POLICIES. One of the most effective ways to prevent risk selection is to make it unprofitable by varying subsidies on the basis of each enrollee's anticipated medical expenses. Known as risk adjustment, this strategy bases subsidies on enrollee characteristics related to the use of health care such as age and past use of health care. Risk adjustment addresses two problems associated with uniform subsidies. First, if subsidies to plans were uniform and insurers could change premiums on the basis of enrollees' characteristics (which is not allowed in Medicare), then sicker and older beneficiaries might not be able to afford coverage. Second, if subsidies were uniform and if insurers had to charge everyone the same premium, then the incentive for plans to enroll those with low anticipated costs or to simply not participate in Medicare would be overwhelming. For these reasons, Medicare policy has long included risk adjustment for private plan payments.

The competition envisioned under premium support hinges on the success of risk adjustment in varying subsidies enough to make risk selection unprofitable. Medicare already varies its payments to health plans in line with patients' age, sex, disability status, Medicaid status, employment status, and past hospitalization experience.[10] But these payment differentials miss much of the variation in actual spending. With the information currently available to them, public authorities can predict only about 25–30 percent of the total variation in annual health care spending.[11] Such calculations could benefit from additional information available to insurers, who can observe enrollees' health status. For example, the risk adjustment system used for the Medicare drug benefit offsets about one-quarter of the variation in outlays but could offset half if past drug usage were included in the formula.[12]

Measures other than risk adjustment could reduce the gains from efforts to attract low-cost patients. Medicare could pay separately for extremely high-cost conditions or treatments, as it does now for unusually lengthy or costly hospital episodes. Such payments directly attenuate the financial consequences for a health plan that "gets stuck with" an unusually costly caseload. Medicare could pay a percentage of claims above some threshold—known as reinsurance—as it does now for plans offering drug benefits under Part D. Medicare could employ "risk corridors" to symmetrically limit potential profits and losses, as it also does for Part D plans. If plan costs exceed target expenses by a certain range, Medicare shares in the losses. If costs are lower than the bottom of the risk corridor, Medicare recaptures part of the savings. So-called carve-outs—or separate payments for specific services—can also protect insurers from very high costs, such as those arising from cancer or senile dementia.

Each of these approaches reduces losses from enrolling high-cost patients. Except for risk adjustment and carve-outs, however, they also reduce incentives to operate efficiently and control costs.

CONSUMER INFORMATION AND MARKETING. Unbiased assistance is essential if enrollees are to select intelligently among insurance offerings. All insurance is complex, health insurance exceedingly so. Health insurance stipulates what charges will be imposed in many situations, including some that are remote, improbable, emotionally troubling, and very important. It also stipulates what rights individuals retain, and what rights they surrender. Implicit in these agreements are the laws of contracts and torts, which few lay people understand. Few people know whether failure to provide an ordinary X-ray, a CT scan, an MRI scan, or a PET scan for persistent bone pain is standard practice or malpractice. They depend on physicians to make these decisions in their interest, but it is physicians whose behaviors may be curbed by constraints that set the terms of their payment. Furthermore, choosing among plans poses special challenges for the mentally or physically infirm, not all of whom have competent relatives or other advisers to assist them.

Under premium support, informing and protecting Medicare beneficiaries in their selection of insurance coverage would not be left solely to insurance companies. Insurers, by definition, are in the business of trying to sell insurance and make profits for shareholders. Their interests are not always aligned with those of their enrollees. As a result, the task of informing potential enrollees about plan characteristics should be performed or supervised by independent third parties—public agencies or private organizations acting as agents for the public. These third parties would collect information from insurers, convey it to potential enrollees, and handle enrollment. They would also provide counseling to those who need it. Insurers would be barred from using insurance agents and door-to-door marketing.

PARTICIPATION RULES. The government would have to set conditions under which health insurers could enter or leave particular health care markets. Without such limits, insurers could create havoc for beneficiaries by entering or leaving on the basis of short-term conditions in that market. This problem would be especially acute where few insurers operate, as in rural areas.

Regulations would also be necessary to discourage enrollees from abusing plans by opting for the cheapest possible plan when healthy and then shifting to the most generous one when sick. Such regulations would specify a minimum period of enrollment and penalties for "premature" cancellation, for example. Medicare now has such policies. People who do not enroll in Parts B and D soon after becoming eligible face higher premiums if they enroll later. Medicare Advantage enrollees generally may leave plans only during periods of open enrollment.

### Selecting and Paying Providers

One of the most effective management tools available to health plans is their ability to include only those providers who agree to abide by the plan's rules. Health plans are unable to promote quality protocols, implement care coordination, and simplify administration through common information technology, for example, without the cooperation of health providers, who typically are reluctant to respond to health plan demands. Getting providers to accept price discounts is an even greater challenge. Plans derive their leverage from being able to deny Medicare payments to uncooperative providers. Thus plans need considerable discretion to exclude providers from approved networks. This power carries risks, however. Plans could avoid contracting with providers who treat high-cost illnesses—cancer or AIDS, for instance. They could locate offices far from areas in which high-cost populations live so as to discourage their enrollment. At best, such policies simply cause patients to switch plans. At worst, they deprive some people of adequate care. To avoid this risk, Medicare would need to ensure that plans offer an adequate roster of health providers. Medicare Advantage and the drug benefit each have network adequacy rules. These rules would have to be strengthened under premium support as there would be no guaranteed fee-for-service alternative.

### How Quality Is Promoted

Advocates of premium support complain that fee-for-service Medicare provides uncoordinated, duplicative, and incomplete care. A patient may seek care from many providers, none of whom may be clearly responsible for the patient's medical outcome. This problem is particularly serious for patients with multiple or chronic conditions, who account for most medical care expenditures. Even if responsibility could be assigned, physician performance would be difficult to evaluate because each provider typically treats too few Medicare patients with any particular condition to support valid statistical inferences. Furthermore, Medicare does not pay physicians to communicate with one another, even if such communication lowers overall costs or improves care.

Competing plans would have both the means and the incentive to insist on such communication. Plans with many Medicare participants can readily collect and compile information on effectiveness and cost. Such information could be used as a management and marketing tool. Coordinated care plans offered under Medicare Advantage already use these methods. Each year the National Committee on Quality Assurance evaluates these plans on the basis of more than forty indicators that are thought to contribute to high-quality care.[13]

Under premium support, the importance of measuring quality and helping enrollees compare plans would increase because all beneficiaries could choose their plans and switch periodically. If even a modest fraction of enrollees were to choose a plan on the basis of such information, insurers would have a strong incentive to maintain high ratings. Because enrollees could switch plans annually, however, the tendency would be to focus on immediate and dramatic improvements—such as procurement of new, high-tech equipment—more than on procedures with long-run implications, such as stopping smoking.

Premium support might also be better equipped to improve quality since private plans have tools that a single-payer system like Medicare would be unlikely to use. Private plans would be less encumbered by political pressures than Medicare is now. They could exclude low-quality providers and select their networks from the pool of physicians, clinics, and hospitals that meet specific practice or cost standards. In addition, they might introduce new technologies and implement new ways of delivering care more rapidly than can a large bureaucracy. Doing so could give them a marketing edge as they compete for enrollees.

## What a Typical Beneficiary Would Encounter

To appreciate how premium support would work, suppose that Ms. Brown is newly eligible for Medicare.[14] Just before she reaches her sixty-fifth birthday, Ms. Brown receives a notice from the government informing her that she is about to become eligible for Medicare premium support. She receives two forms, one for her physician to fill out certifying her medical conditions and one for her to fill out to enroll in Medicare.

On the basis of the physician's responses, the Medicare agency places Ms. Brown in a particular "risk class," which in turn determines the subsidy that will be paid to any plan she selects. The subsidy will depend on the average cost of providing a given set of benefits to that class and thus will differ from one risk class to another. In other words, everyone in a given risk class will receive the same subsidy, and everyone, regardless of risk class, will face the same charge for enrolling in any given plan.

With her subsidy in hand, Ms. Brown chooses among alternative qualifying plans offered in her community. The plan offerings will differ in their premiums, provider networks, quality ratings, and extra services. If the plan Ms. Brown chooses provides Medicare benefits at a price lower than the local risk-adjusted benchmark, she will receive supplemental benefits or a rebate in the form of a lower premium. If the plan's price exceeds the benchmark, she will have to pay an additional premium equal to the difference. Ms. Brown's premium will increase in this way to cover the added costs of extra coverage, lower deductibles, a broader network of providers, or a less efficient plan. If Ms. Brown has retiree health coverage from a former employer, the employer could apply its contribution to her Medicare premium. If Ms. Brown is poor, either Medicaid or Medicare will provide an additional subsidy to cover premiums, deductibles, coinsurance, and additional services, much as Medicaid does now.

Ms. Brown receives information on her plan choices from an organization independent of the plans but sponsored by Medicare. She applies for benefits either at the organization's offices, the local Medicare office, or on the Internet. She can bring a relative, friend, or adviser with her to help her make sense of the information that she receives. Government-financed counseling is also available.

Once Ms. Brown is enrolled, she has to remain with her plan for one year. During that time, her premium and subsidy are fixed. At the end of a year, Ms. Brown is free to change plans during an "open enrollment" period lasting perhaps thirty days. The plan may also be allowed to revise premiums, benefits, and its network of providers. The government adjusts the subsidy Ms. Brown receives for both the growth of health care expenditures and any change in her risk status.

If Ms. Brown is healthy at enrollment, she might choose a plan with a low premium but high cost sharing. Such a plan would be financially manageable if her good health continued. Should her health deteriorate, she might regret her choice. Suppose that at the age of sixty-six she has a heart attack. Almost all private plans have good hospital coverage. However, she will have to pay her full, relatively high deductible for the first day of her hospitalization. In addition, she might not be able to see the cardiologist of her choice if she has selected a low-cost plan with a tight provider network. She will have no chance to choose a new plan until the end of her annual enrollment period.

How Ms. Brown would fare under premium support if she developed a chronic illness is hard to predict. Say that at the age of sixty-seven she develops lower back pain. Her doctor lists three treatment options: back surgery, medication, or physical therapy. Her insurance plan, which has a financial incentive to return her to health, assigns Ms. Brown a care coordinator. This person ensures that Ms. Brown receives disease management and prescription drugs. The surgery will be covered by the plan—but only after she exhausts the therapies suggested by the care coordinator. The plan does not cover physical therapy since that benefit tends to attract enrollees with disabilities. In brief, Ms. Brown would benefit from the incentives that private plans have to keep her healthy but could have less choice about her care and could have no coverage if that illness borders on a disability.

## The Devilish Details

Premium support plans can vary significantly. These differences reflect disagreement over several key aspects of plan design.

### *Specificity of the Benefits Package*

How broad or narrow would benefits be? Tight legislative control of the benefit package has been resisted by premium support advocates because it would impose uniformity and could hamper measures to limit cost. Suppose that a plan were permitted to require screening for mental health services by a psychiatric social worker before patients could see a psychiatrist. Such a requirement could curtail inappropriate use of expensive care, saving money that could be better spent elsewhere. Or, to the extent that mental and somatic illnesses are positively correlated, it may serve to discourage high-cost patients from joining the plan. How benefits are defined could determine whether the proposal limits access—or discourages innovation.

Policy regarding supplemental coverage is equally important. If Medicare continues to cover only a portion of its beneficiaries' health care spending, the demand for supplemental benefits will persist. Standardizing supplemental benefits makes it easier for beneficiaries to compare alternative plans and to buy the one that best matches their wants, but it carries the risk that some may not find a plan that meets their particular needs and is contrary to the spirit of premium support. Finding the right balance between flexibility and simplicity is a central challenge.

## *How Subsidies Are Set*

Because premium support would delegate most of Medicare's current functions to insurers, its primary policy tool would be how it pays those insurers. Payments would have to be sufficient to ensure beneficiaries' access to health plans, but not so high as to defeat the objective of cost control. The version of premium support that uses regional benchmarks is predicated on the expectation that competition will produce this balance. That said, if plan competition does not achieve the intended result, Medicare costs will rise unabated since there are no other checks or balances in the system.

Geographic variation in cost poses another large and politically explosive challenge to premium support. Current Medicare expenditures vary because prices, practice patterns, and the incidence of disease differ from place to place. At present, Medicare beneficiaries pay the same premium and deductibles regardless of variations in spending per enrollee. Consequently, Medicare spends far more per enrollee in high-cost areas than in low-cost areas. This variability has drawn complaints from elected officials in low-cost areas. Because premium support would make these cross-subsidies explicit and clear to all, areas with lower-than-average subsidies would be bound to challenge the system's fairness and press to narrow those differences. If policymakers provided nationally uniform subsidies, the opposite problem would emerge. Enrollees in different areas would pay widely varying out-of-pocket costs for the same coverage, and those in high-cost areas would challenge the fairness of paying more for the same services than other enrollees do. This issue would be a formidable political obstacle to the adoption of premium support.

## *Picking an Approach to Risk Adjustment*

Under premium support, Medicare subsidies would clearly have to be risk adjusted. What remains unclear is whether additional measures to protect plans from losses generated by high-cost enrollees would be necessary to discourage risk selection. The Medicare drug benefit provides reinsurance for catastrophic costs but also protects plans from aggregate costs outside risk corridors. Although universal enrollment may obviate the need for protection against outliers, without such safeguards plans may be reluctant to participate, narrow their offerings, and boost their bids for fear of getting stuck with high-cost enrollees. Retroactive reimbursement would provide full risk adjustment but would re-create the current system with its cost-increasing incentives. The difference between full and no exposure to risk could be split by combining prospective payment with partial payment based on actual costs, but striking the right balance is difficult.

## Assessment

Advocates of premium support believe that it will merge the best features of social insurance with market competition. It relies on competing private insurers rather than Congress to set provider payment rates. It aligns Medicare's delivery system organization with that used by employers. It balances assurances of coverage with incentives for efficiency and quality. By delegating decisions to private insurers, it is less subject to lobbying and politics than traditional Medicare, where even collecting data on quality is politically charged because providers fear that Medicare will use the information against them. And it would do away with the current hodgepodge of overlapping supplemental coverage plans. In the decade since the concept emerged, experience with managed care—in general and in Medicare—has shed some light on the model's potential to achieve Medicare's goals of access, quality improvement, and cost control.

### Ensuring Access

In theory, Medicare's subsidies to private plans and benefit rules should ensure access comparable to that under the current program. Access would improve if beneficiaries, accurately anticipating their own needs, enrolled in plans that met them. Furthermore, because plans have an incentive to hold down costs, they may lower cost sharing for services such as prevention and maintenance drugs, thereby improving access to them.

Practically speaking, however, premium support may have difficulty fulfilling this promise for at least two important reasons. First, Medicare may be unable to adjust payments enough to discourage plans from competing to attract low-cost enrollees. Insurance markets are plagued by incomplete information. Actual or potential enrollees usually know more about their own health and their likely use of health care services than do the companies that sell them insurance. If risk adjustment fails to neutralize self-selection by high-cost enrollees, companies could adopt policies to discourage their enrollment. They might limit the number of providers in the networks or reduce payment rates, thereby curtailing patients' access to the providers of their choice. Plans might impose procedural barriers to care such as preapproval for the use of expensive drugs. They could also design benefits so as to shed high-risk enrollees. Lowering cost sharing for low-cost care while raising it for high-cost care might improve access for healthy enrollees but would reduce it for sick enrollees, who need access the most. As research has shown, enrollees of managed care plans appear to have lower access than do those in other types of plans.[15]

Second, premium support, like other market-oriented health models (see chapter 6), assumes that Medicare consumers supplied with clear information and financial incentives will choose a plan that best meets their needs. In fact, most potential enrollees do not have enough information, time, or skill to evaluate products as complex as health insurance policies. A significant fraction of Medicare beneficiaries have multiple, chronic conditions, suffer from a mental illness or impairment, have low education and income, or some other characteristic that makes assessing one's own needs challenging. Even well-educated and unimpaired beneficiaries have difficulty choosing plans wisely. An important body of behavioral economics research documents that people are not good at anticipating their preferences under unanticipated or new circumstances and that they sometimes consider choices they themselves have made to be inferior.[16] A mismatch between health needs and plan design would diminish access as well as satisfaction.

## Promoting Quality and Satisfaction

The enormous variation in the quality of health care under Medicare, as in the entire health system, is well documented. Medicare has done more to monitor quality in its private plans than in the traditional program. To date, however, there is little or no evidence that the quality of care provided by health maintenance organizations or other organized health plans for beneficiaries differs materially and systematically from that offered by traditional Medicare.[17] Most physicians, nursing homes, hospitals, and other providers serve patients regardless of their plan. Since provider practice generally does not vary with the patient's insurance coverage, people enrolled in Medicare Advantage, traditional fee-for-service Medicare, and employer-sponsored plans typically receive comparable care.[18]

Some of the tools that managed care plans use to promote quality conflict with the goal of maintaining satisfaction among enrollees. Many potential enrollees seem more interested in the obvious convenience of a wide choice of nearby providers than in hard-to-observe quality measures.[19] Plans have thus expanded their networks well beyond the limits that would allow them to coordinate care effectively and exclude low-quality providers. Moreover, few plans have made quality the dominant consideration in selecting network providers, as the best physicians and hospitals are in high demand and therefore less likely than other providers to accept the offer of discounted payments that plans bent on controlling costs are willing to offer. This situation might well change, however, if all Medicare patients were enrolled in competing plans.

Another factor to consider is that, in some respects, premium support offers less choice than other models. Although traditional Medicare offers no choice in the core benefit package, it provides enrollees with unlimited choice among physicians, hospitals, and other providers. Premium support would offer an expanded range of insurance options. But if plans manage care aggressively, they would perforce restrict the choice of providers. And, as a practical matter, the benefit packages in a premium support system may not vary greatly. The various plans offered under the Federal Employees Health Benefit system, which is often held up as a model for a competitive Medicare system, closely resemble one another. Most participants seem to want roughly the same coverage, which raises a question about the much-vaunted welfare gains from matching insurance to allegedly diverse tastes. Which form of choice produces better quality gains is not clear. As far as patient satisfaction goes, it seems that patients are happier when given a choice of providers than they are when given a choice of plans.[20]

## Controlling Costs

According to its advocates, premium support would lower the rate of growth and possibly the level of Medicare spending because plans would become more efficient and reduce waste in their efforts to attract enrollees. Because Medicare's payments to them would be capped, insurers would want to control spending. The ability of private plans to employ a number of tools not easily adopted by Medicare—for example, closed drug formularies, limited provider networks, variable cost sharing—provides the means. Cost-conscious health plans, it is claimed, would invest in wellness programs and care management to avoid preventable illness and costs. Insurers would set formularies and coverage rules that heighten incentives for drug and device companies to develop cost-reducing, as well as quality-increasing, therapies. And provider fees would, theoretically, be lower than

Medicare's administratively set rates because plans could set rates competitively and restrict networks. On the demand side, forcing enrollees to bear the cost of premiums above what the government pays would heighten cost consciousness. Beneficiaries would have economic incentives to look for plans that weigh benefits against costs and offer low-cost and high-quality providers. Enrollees would also pay more for, and use less of, the services that plans deem to be of lower value. For all these reasons, premium support would likely lower the overall cost of providing health care to Medicare beneficiaries.

Arguably, savings would come more from curtailing use than from cutting prices. The various ways that a plan can limit use are both less obvious and important in marketing to enrollees than those they have to limit price. To attract enrollees, some plans would likely construct networks that include popular, high-quality—and high-price—providers. In fact, physician payment rates of private plans in 2006 were about 20 percent higher than fees traditional Medicare paid.[21] Similarly, marketing may force plans to cover the newest tests, technology, and drugs irrespective of their marginal benefit. Marketing costs themselves would rise, adding to premiums. Indeed, the aggressive use of benefit rules and the ability to design coverage would probably make it easier to lower use than to lower price.

While premium support would probably slow the growth of total spending, its impact on federal spending seems less clear. Preliminary experience with drug plans under Part D suggests that insurers price their plans near what they think the benchmarks will be, allowing for some premium rebates or additional benefits but doing little to hold down federal costs. Such collusive behavior, if sustained, drives up benchmarks, causing Medicare to pay for an increasing fraction of its beneficiaries' health care over time, as it indirectly subsidizes supplemental coverage.[22]

In view of the uncertainty of premium support's impact on federal spending, those charged with estimating the costs of Medicare proposals have been slow to conclude that this system would produce large immediate savings or significantly reduce the growth of spending. According to estimates of Medicare's Office of the Actuary, the annual growth of Medicare spending would run about a half a percentage point lower over the first decade of a premium support plan like the one proposed by the Medicare Commission in 1999 than it would under the current program.[23] The staff of the commission was more "bullish" on potential savings, estimating a reduction in Medicare spending growth of about 1 percentage point a year over the first decade.[24] When the Congressional Budget Office examined different options for structuring premium support in 2006, it found that reductions in federal spending might be achieved, but only if Medicare spending were linked to an index that grows less than health care spending.[25]

In arguing that premium support helps the government better control its budget, the model's advocates risk abandoning the chief advantage they claim over traditional voucher plans. Because payments to plans would be based on actual health care costs, premium support could sustain something akin to a defined benefit with a defined contribution. This linkage would reduce the likelihood of federal savings. For this reason, liberal critics of premium support fear that Congress, which continually faces difficult budgetary tradeoffs, would stint on annual increases in the premium subsidy.[26] The result, they argue, could easily be a slow-motion repeal of Medicare's protections, even if the benefits package remained officially unchanged. Congress could simply ratchet down the rate at which payments to private plans are increased, leaving to insurers the task of figuring out how to cut use, fees, or both. In the end, the proposition that premium support would lower federal Medicare spending or slow its growth retains considerable theoretical appeal, but realizing those savings will depend on how the program is designed and implemented.

## Conclusion

Premium support is one of the few major ideas for Medicare that has moved from theory into practice. It inspired the design of the Medicare drug benefit and is the principle underlying Medicare Advantage. A premium support demonstration designed to promote competition between Medicare Advantage plans and traditional Medicare is slated to go into effect in 2010. If current trends continue, an increasing proportion of Medicare beneficiaries will enroll in private plans. The "carrots" that are boosting enrollment in the current system could be supplemented by "sticks" to move all beneficiaries into private plans (for example, new beneficiaries could be prohibited from enrolling in fee-for-service Medicare). If the system is introduced gradually, the difficult political and analytical choices required to make it work might meet with less resistance. Alternatively, premium support could be enacted as part of legislation to reform Medicare, to address its financing crisis, or to reform other parts of the health care system.

All versions of premium support rest on the assumption that private plans can organize and pay for health care for Medicare beneficiaries better than the government or individuals can. It would blend regulation designed to ensure access with competition designed to lower costs and raise quality. It also has the appeal of a public-private partnership—a hybrid of public funding and rules, on one hand, and private delivery and innovation, on the other. However, the design of premium support is as important as its theory in determining whether it will ensure access, improve quality, and control costs. A fully implemented premium support system designed to address any limitations could succeed at reducing overall health costs and possibly Medicare costs, but this could come at the price of reduced access and limited improvements in quality.

# 6 Consumer-Directed Medicare

U nder consumer-directed health care, decisionmaking rests with individuals, not with the government (as in social insurance) or with health plans (as in premium support). People would pay for health care through accounts linked to high-deductible insurance plans. This reform springs from the concept of the "ownership society," in which much of the responsibility for education, pensions, and health care would be shifted from the government to individuals.[1] In the case of education, for example, parents would send their children to schools they chose and pay tuition with vouchers the government gave them. People would finance their retirement from individually owned savings accounts into which they would deposit all or part of their Social Security payroll taxes. And a consumer-directed model would replace the traditional Medicare program.

In this model, high-deductible insurance coverage would be coupled with personal accounts for out-of-pocket spending. The accounts would be seeded with Medicare funding that a social insurance program would otherwise have used to pay providers directly or that premium support would have funneled to health plans. The deposit would be larger for low-income than for high-income beneficiaries. These subsidized accounts could be used to pay a wide range of health care providers for an equally broad menu of services. Each person would have the responsibility to learn about the prices and quality of care offered in the medical marketplace. Insurers would guarantee a limit on out-of-pocket spending. They might also provide enrollees with tools to navigate the system. Insurance plans would be free to seek discounts through provider networks or formularies and could implement programs to promote disease management or prevention or to improve quality, but these services are not integral to the approach.

The consumer-directed model would sharply increase the range of health care decisions made by individuals themselves rather than collectively through social insurance or by insurers. The services covered by high-deductible plans would be loosely defined. Individuals would decide how to use their personal accounts. Supporters also argue that this alternative would give consumers the incentive to use only needed care and to shop frugally. If health care spending were low, account balances would grow.[2] A presumed increase in consumer price sensitivity would cause providers to curb needless use of costly procedures. This shift in incentives would allegedly dampen the "medical arms race" that results from consumer price insensitivity induced by insurance with low deductibles.

The system's advocates view Medicare as a glaring example of a "nanny state" that pays even for small outlays and thus deludes beneficiaries into believing that health care is free or nearly free. They also complain that Medicare's undifferentiated benefits package does not accommodate the diverse insurance preferences of individuals. Critics of consumer-directed health care, in contrast, claim that its advocates overstate its benefits and understate the risk that it would reduce access to care and increase financial hardship for low-income and sick beneficiaries.

To explain how consumer-directed Medicare would work, we examine the Bush administration's medical savings account demonstration. Implemented in 2007, this demonstration allows people with high-deductible health plans to receive Medicare contributions in savings accounts.[3]

## Origins

Consumer-directed health care rests on a well-developed political philosophy that embraces private means of production and distribution and free markets.[4] Societal goals are said to be best achieved through individual rather than collective action. In health care, for example, individuals empowered through accounts and information are expected to make decisions that yield higher welfare than would result from government intervention. This view reflects a traditional American belief that people excel when they are liberated from bureaucratic restrictions and permitted to guide their own destinies and that government programs such as Medicare deny free choice and undermine personal responsibility.

Proponents of this form of market competition believe that individuals' own behavior drives and can hold down health care spending. They note that more than three-fourths of spending now derives from chronic illness, and claim that much of that spending could be prevented or managed by individuals through behavioral changes and appropriate and early use of health care.[5] If people had a larger stake in the cost of their care, they might smoke or overeat less or seek health care that staves off illness and saves money.

This view also reflects the libertarian emphasis on consumer control, unfettered by restrictions imposed externally by the government or by insurance companies. Both libertarians and social conservatives believe that government involvement in health care stifles innovation. The former deplore any interference with personal moral decisions concerning life and death.[6] The National Right to Life Committee, for one, has been a staunch supporter of private health plans with few restrictions, fearing that the government or managed care plans would try to save money by disallowing costly life-prolonging treatments.[7] Fiscal conservatives support consumer-directed health care also because they believe it will restrain government spending and interference in economic and social life. Consumer-directed health care has found some support among medical practitioners exasperated by the layers of payment rules and regulations that stand between them and their patients and interfere with the practice of medicine.[8]

The consumer-directed model evolved from "medical savings accounts" (MSAs), which are tax-preferred saving accounts that can be used to pay for premiums and cost sharing linked to high-deductible health insurance plans. MSAs became the conservatives' alternative to President Bill Clinton's comprehensive reform plan debated in 1994.[9] When the Clinton plan failed, MSAs became a part of the 1995 Republican Medicare reform plan, Medisave.[10] This proposal failed as well.

Although President Clinton was opposed to a national MSA policy, he accepted MSA pilot demonstrations for the working population in 1996 and for the Medicare population in 1997. The 1996 demonstration allowed up to 750,000 policies with deductibles of at least $1,500. Account deposits were limited to 65 percent of the deductible. They could be sold only to people who had no access to employer-sponsored insurance. The Medicare demonstration would have allowed 390,000 people to enroll in plans with a minimum deductible of $6,000 per year, no cost sharing above the deductible, and a Medicare account deposit equal to the difference between the area's capitation rate and the plan's premium for the high-deductible plan. Neither of the demonstrations proved popular with insurers or potential enrollees. Only about 250,000 nonelderly families—less than one-third of the cap—ever reported having an MSA before the demonstration ended in 2001.[11] No plan offered a Medicare MSA under the original demonstration authority.

Consumer-directed health care received a major policy boost in 2003 with passage of the Medicare Modernization Act (MMA). Before the MMA, congressional Republicans were divided on the approach. The leadership had embraced an insurance-based premium support plan to deliver the drug benefit and administer the managed care part of Medicare. Many conservatives preferred consumer direction over premium support, which in their view fostered big government and HMOs. To gain the support of conservatives, the final bill permanently authorized consumer-directed plans for both the nonelderly and Medicare beneficiaries.[12]

For the nonelderly, this option took the form of Health Savings Accounts (HSAs). These reincarnated MSAs allow anyone who buys a high-deductible health plan (with deductibles of at least $1,100 for individuals and $2,200 for couples or families in 2008) to create a tax-favored HSA. HSAs now receive more favorable tax treatment than is granted any other form of saving. Deposits are not subject to personal income or payroll taxes. Investment earnings are similarly exempt. And withdrawals used for health care are also tax free. Withdrawals for purposes other than health care are taxed as ordinary income plus a 10 percent penalty tax. The penalty is waived, however, in cases of disability or death or for individuals age 65 or over.[13] Unused balances remain available forever and keep generating tax-free investment income until used.[14] An HSA option was also introduced into the Federal Employees Health Benefits System in January 2005. As of 2006, only about 7,500 of the roughly 9 million federal employees and dependents eligible to participate enrolled in these consumer-directed health plans.[15]

The MMA also added a new, unlimited MSA option to Medicare Advantage. Medicare beneficiaries who buy a plan with a maximum deductible of $10,500 in 2008 receive a Medicare contribution to an account. The contribution is based on the plan's risk-adjusted bid plus the difference between the standardized local Medicare Advantage benchmark and the plan's bid if the benchmark is higher (which is almost always the case). There is no cost sharing for Medicare-covered services above the deductible, but plans cannot waive the deductible for Medicare-covered preventive or other services.[16] Like other Medicare Advantage plans but unlike traditional Medicare, the plans may establish a preferred network of providers. They can neither restrict enrollees to these networks nor establish different cost-sharing amounts for services received from in-network and out-of-network providers. No such plans were offered in 2006. As a result, in the summer of 2006 the administration proposed a demonstration for the following year that gave insurers the flexibility to offer plans similar to the high-deductible HSAs available in the non-Medicare market.[17] By the end of 2007, 2,271 beneficiaries had enrolled in two standard MSAs, with none opting for the lone demonstration plan. No demonstration plan was offered in 2008, although standard MSAs became available nationwide and attracted about 3,300 beneficiaries to one of nine plans.[18] Proposals to expand consumer-directed health care in Medicare were introduced in Congress subsequent to implementation of the MMA, but chances for enactment evaporated with the change to a Democratic majority in 2007.[19]

## How Consumer-Directed Medicare Would Work

Under a consumer-directed system, Medicare's subsidy would consist of a payment for high-deductible insurance and a deposit in beneficiaries' personal accounts. Medicare would operate as a true defined-contribution program rather than a defined-benefit one. In contrast to social insurance and premium support, consumer-directed Medicare would directly reward beneficiaries for efficient and discriminating use of care—but would leave them at risk if the account or insurance plan were inadequate.

Consumer-directed Medicare could take many forms but would likely have several distinct features. It would partially subsidize health insurance plans, cap annual out-of-pocket payments, and provide enrollees with tools to navigate the system. The plans could, but would not necessarily, seek discounts through provider networks or formularies, implement programs to promote disease management or prevention, or use market leverage to improve quality. The personal accounts would be seeded with funds that would have been used to pay providers under social insurance or health plans under premium support. Beneficiaries could use the subsidized accounts for a wide range of health care providers and services. Beneficiaries would be responsible for determining how much and what kinds of care they seek. Key plan variables include the level of the deductible and out-of-pocket maximum, whether deductibles can be waived for some services, the amounts to be contributed to the accounts, and whether the account balances could be used for non-health purposes. In this chapter, we assume consumer-directed Medicare would resemble the MSA demonstration project proposed in 2006 by the Bush administration, a leading champion of this model of health care.[20]

### High-Deductible Health Plans

Medicare would no longer pay for health care directly. Private, high-deductible health insurance plans and beneficiaries would do so. Beneficiaries would enroll in such plans much as they now enroll in a drug or Medicare Advantage plan. A minimum deductible would be set by law or regulation.[21] In 2008 annual deductibles offered to beneficiaries in standard MSAs ranged from $2,500 to $5,100 per person.[22] This minimum deductible would be adjusted annually in line with the growth of health care spending.

Once expenses equal the deductible, insurance would cover most additional outlays. To keep beneficiaries aware of total health care spending and discourage overuse, plans would require the insured person to pay a small portion of costs—say, 10–15 percent—above the deductible until some out-of-pocket maximum is reached. In the demonstration, the catastrophic limit for qualified health spending in 2008 was $10,500.[23] Plans would also have the option, currently available under HSAs, to cover preventive care and selected services with no deductible.

The actuarial value of services covered and account subsidies would approximate that of current Medicare coverage. Plans would have wide flexibility in determining covered benefits. For example, they could scale back coverage of one benefit to increase coverage of another.

Whether such high-deductible plans would work to control service price and use is unclear. High-deductible health plans would cover a smaller fraction of expenditures than Medicare now does. This feature would reduce their ability—and interest—in developing provider networks and negotiating discounts. However, they would offer stop-loss coverage, and this feature would expose them to unlimited liability, a consideration that would heighten interest in constraining outlays during at least very-high-cost episodes.

Historically, consumer-directed health insurance has not offered group discounts. A few plans have used discounts negotiated in the group market to attract individual customers. A key factor in evaluating this proposal is whether plan savings flow from price discounts or from reduced use of services, some of which are highly beneficial.

### The Personal Account

All beneficiaries would have a high-deductible health plan linked to a personal bank account. Banks would offer a menu of investment options. Medicare would deposit a lump sum into the account annually. Beneficiaries could also contribute to this account, as long as the total annual contributions from Medicare and beneficiaries amount to at least $500 less than the deductible. Unspent personal account balances would accrue interest tax-free. With carryovers, account balances could exceed deductibles. If the account were depleted, beneficiaries would not receive additional account deposits from Medicare until the following year. And they would not be allowed to borrow against future deposits. Beneficiaries could use the personal account balances for medical purposes, including services not covered by the high-deductible plan such as dental care, vision care, guide-dog services, home improvements for people with disabilities, certain foods for medical diets, and wigs for people who have lost their hair because of disease.[24] Use of funds for nonmedical purposes would trigger a tax penalty.

If enrollees receive useful information on health care services, chances are greater that consumer-directed Medicare will work as intended. Price information would be available in two ways. The high-deductible insurance plans would give enrollees access to information on any price discounts that they might negotiate with providers for costs beneficiaries incur under the deductible. The Medicare MSA demonstration follows this policy, as do Medicare drug plans and many commercial consumer-directed health plans.[25] Medicare could also create systemwide requirements for price transparency from providers. For example, doctors or hospitals that serve seniors could be required to post price information. Additional quality reporting would reduce any confusion and fraud that could occur when Medicare's payment systems are replaced by individuals purchasing services directly.

The central principle of all such plans is that people should be provided with the means to buy care but should be required to face the reality that funds spent on health care today reduce one's capacity to consume health care or anything else later. Roughly half of Medicare beneficiaries spent less than $2,000 in 2008.[26] A personal account deposit of $2,000 would therefore cover all health care costs for roughly half of all beneficiaries. This fraction might increase if, as advocates anticipate, high-deductible health insurance causes people to cut spending. Beneficiaries who spend less than is deposited in their accounts would pocket the savings. On the other hand, enrollees who spend more than the personal account balance would be fully exposed to those costs, plus charges for uncovered services.

## Medicare Payments to Accounts and Plans

Medicare payments would be divided between deposits to individual accounts and payment of insurance premiums. The government would calculate a regional payment benchmark.[27] Each plan would calculate a "bid"—the price at which it would sell a high-deductible plan in a region. The bid would be below the benchmark because high-deductible coverage costs less than comprehensive coverage, which is the basis of the regional payment benchmark. Each plan would deposit the difference between the Medicare payment for the regional benchmark and the plan bid in the enrollees' personal accounts. All enrollees in each plan would receive the same Medicare-subsidized account deposit. The deposit would not be permitted to exceed the deductible less $500.[28] Medicare's payments to high-deductible plans would be risk-adjusted to discourage cherry-picking by insurers.

The proposal's long-term budget implications will depend largely on how the benchmark is updated. Annual increases would presumably be linked to some index since system supporters envision predictable, fixed costs over time. An index such as the change in per capita income or the gross domestic product (GDP) would keep public spending on Medicare in line with those economic indicators. Medicare's spending would rise or fall as a share of national income only as the share of the population eligible for Medicare changes.

Alternatively, the index used to adjust the benchmark could be related to the growth of per capita private health care spending, which varies widely from year to year.[29] For example, real per capita private health care spending actually fell 0.5 percent in 1994, grew 6.3 percent in 2002, and slowed to 1.2 percent growth in 2006.[30] Because the growth of Medicare costs has historically tracked that of private health spending, this approach would be unlikely to reduce projected spending materially unless it reduced the growth of health care spending on the general population. Annual spending adjustments would be smaller on average and would vary less if they were linked to changes in personal income or GDP.

*Quality Systems and Provider Choice*

As already mentioned, the core principle underlying consumer-directed Medicare is that people should bear increased responsibility for their own medical decisions. Medicare or other government agencies might provide information on quality or prices, but beneficiaries, guided by appropriate financial incentives, would weigh those and other factors and then decide which providers to patronize. Patients with high blood pressure, for example, could buy expensive, brand-name drugs without interference from an insurer if they thought those medications were worth the cost. They could buy less costly and, perhaps, less effective drugs that seemed to them to be better value for the money. Or they could opt for a regimen of diet control and exercise and forgo drug treatment altogether. Patients have such options now, but insurance shields them and their providers from the financial implications of their choices. Under consumer-directed, high-deductible insurance, they would directly confront such consequences. The result, advocates believe, would be an increase in demand for cost-effective care that providers would compete to supply.

Information on quality, as well as on prices, is essential to the effective functioning of the consumer-directed model. More than they do now, beneficiaries would need to know what therapies and which therapists work best because they, not Medicare or insurers, would be responsible for selecting providers and would face increased financial consequences of their medical decisions. Numerous sources of information on medical therapies have emerged, including WebMD (a computer-based guide to therapies and diseases), Consumer Report's Best Buy Drugs (a comparison of drug prices and effectiveness), and reports of the Agency for Healthcare Research and Quality. If 44 million Americans became responsible for buying their own health care services, the volume of this information—as well as advertising and other forms of marketing—would expand greatly.

A key question for consumer-directed Medicare is who will generate and ensure the accuracy of such information. Those who offer consumer-directed health products routinely provide quality information. Unfortunately, access to it is poor and few enrollees use it.[31] Under the new system, providers would likely advertise and use other means to sell their services. While the government would have a smaller role in regulating health care quality, it would have greater responsibility for ensuring the adequacy and accuracy of information for the new decisionmakers, namely, the beneficiaries.

## *Supplemental Insurance*

Most current Medicare enrollees have supplemental insurance of some kind. Yet a policy that permitted supplemental policies to fill in the high deductible under a consumer-directed health care model would undercut the goal of heightening enrollees' cost sensitivity and boost program costs. For that reason, supplemental coverage could be sold by the same company that supplies catastrophic coverage, but it could not fully fill in the deductible. Beneficiaries would be able to buy supplemental insurance from other vendors for services that are not covered by the high-deductible plan, such as long-term care. Such coverage could be financed by account balances.

## *Systems for Low-Income and Other Special Groups of Beneficiaries*

Medicare beneficiaries with few assets and low incomes currently qualify for special programs that pay for some or all premiums, deductibles, other cost sharing, and some services not covered by Medicare, most notably long-term nursing home care. Patients enrolled in both Medicare and Medicaid—so-called dual-eligibles—are prohibited from participating in the current consumer-directed health care demonstration. In a plan covering all of Medicare, a way would have to be found to retain supplemental benefits for poor enrollees. The current programs could continue, wrapping around the new benefit design (as is assumed in chapters 4 and 5). Or Medicare could lower the deductible or raise the contribution to personal accounts to cover much or all of costs up to the deductible, or even up to the plan's stop-loss limit for vulnerable beneficiaries. Premium assistance would be needed as well, although, as with prescription drug plans, this assistance would likely be reduced if eligible beneficiaries chose high-cost plans. Medicaid would still be needed for services not covered by the high-deductible plans.

Enrollees who are unable to navigate the health care system without assistance present quite different problems. About 7 million, or 16 percent, of beneficiaries qualify for Medicare because of disability. About 5 percent of beneficiaries live in long-term care facilities and more than a quarter have a cognitive or mental impairment. Nearly one-third have less than a high school education.[32] Some are unable to direct their own care. Case managers or personal assistance attendants could be retained for beneficiaries who need assistance in managing their own care. Alternatively, family members, friends, local advocacy organizations, or health providers could be paid to perform these tasks.[33] Some specialized plans could be included that maintain consumer direction but have simplified information, choices, and systems designed for beneficiaries with special needs.[34] Additional payments would be required to ensure plan participation and the availability of supplemental services. In addition, a system of default enrollment in such plans may be needed to prevent vulnerable beneficiaries from falling through the cracks.

## What a Typical Beneficiary Would Encounter

Beneficiaries nearing the age of eligibility for Medicare would receive letters informing them that they will be eligible for a government-subsidized, high-deductible health insurance policy and a lump-sum deposit in a personal account. Suppose one such letter goes to Ms. Brown, a widow living on her deceased husband's Social Security benefits of $18,000 a year. The letter informs Ms. Brown that the insurance will pay for all services now covered by Medicare, but only after she has spent $2,000 in a given year on these services. However, preventative services may be excluded from the deductible and the plan will make a deposit to a personal account that Ms. Brown can use to pay the deductible or other medical expenses. She can choose from several high-deductible health plans that offer coverage in her area. Each plan has a different premium, cost sharing above the deductible, and cap on out-of-pocket expenses. Each will deposit a different amount in a personal account that she may use to pay for health expenses below the out-of-pocket maximum and not covered by the insurance.

After reviewing her choices, Ms. Brown chooses a plan with 10 percent coinsurance above a $2,000 deductible, an out-of-pocket limit of $5,000, and an account deposit of $1,500, the maximum deposit allowed. The plan has an open provider network. It gives Ms. Brown a choice of financial institutions to manage her account. She may invest unused balances in an index stock market fund, a bond fund, or a money market fund. She selects the bond fund, concluding that "bonds are pretty safe" but yield more than the money market fund does. She is healthy and does not expect to spend as much as $1,500 on health care during her first year of eligibility. Still, she is cautious and does not want to take a chance that stock prices might fall.

As it happens, Ms. Brown does stay healthy. In each of her first two years on the plan, she spends only $300—for a physical and a mammogram. She decides not to get a flu shot because she thinks it is not worth the cost: $20 for the vaccine and $50 for the fee of a nurse practitioner. She earns $100 in investment income on the unspent balance, leaving her with a year-end balance in year one of $1,300. Because of inflation, the Medicare benchmark goes up enough to permit the plan to deposit $1,700 at the start of year two, resulting in a start-of-year balance of $3,000.[35] Bond prices rise and, together with interest earnings, Ms. Brown's total investment income is $300 on her enlarged balance. She ends year two with an account balance of $3,000, net of her spending. Now her personal account contains enough to cover not only her deductible but also additional cost sharing that she might face above the deductible. Or she may use some of her personal account to pay for health care services not covered by Medicare, such as dental care.

But Ms. Brown might not be so lucky. Instead of two years of health, she might have a major heart attack soon after she turns sixty-five, might be hospitalized, and undergo coronary artery surgery. Her doctor recommends that after her discharge, she have thirty-six rehabilitative therapy visits. The doctor also prescribes a cholesterol-lowering drug, atorvastatin, which retails for $1,000 a year.[36] Her open-network plan was unable to negotiate discounts from the hospital or surgeon. As a result, the cost of the hospitalization was $75,000, which far exceeds her annual deductible and empties her personal account. She hits her annual out-of-pocket limit of $5,000 while in the hospital. She notes, with relief, that her plan completely covers the cost of her prescription drug. Had she joined a plan with a policy of paying only for the least costly drug in each drug class, she would have had to pay $600 out of pocket for the drug her doctor prescribed because the least costly cholesterol-reducing statin, lovastatin, costs only $400 a year. She is not so fortunate on the rehabilitation, as her plan covers only ten visits. Because her income is modest and rehabilitation visits cost $80 each, Ms. Brown stops therapy after twenty visits, having spent $800 out-of-pocket. In total, she spends $5,800 out of pocket minus the $1,500 account deposit, for a net outlay of $4,300. In her second year, she switches to a plan that covers rehabilitation therapy but gets a lower account deposit of $1,000 as a result.

Many other scenarios are possible. Suppose that during her first year on Medicare, Ms. Brown develops lower back pain from a herniated lumbar disc that causes pressure on a nerve resulting in weakness in her leg that threatens permanent damage if not relieved. Three treatments are available. Back surgery holds the promise of completely relieving pain and avoiding permanent weakness, but it costs $55,000. A steroid injection would relieve pain and temporarily reduce swelling at a cost of $1,050 but might have to be repeated periodically. Physical therapy and pain medication would provide some pain relief at a cost of $700, but offers only a slight chance of a long-term solution. If she chooses surgery, Ms. Brown will spend her entire account, plus $3,500 of her own funds, on cost sharing before the out-of-pocket limit is reached. Her modest income makes this unaffordable. She struggles to choose between the two less costly options. Is the effort and discomfort of physical therapy worth the $350 she would save by forgoing an injection? Under either scenario, she has enough in her account to pay for this care. She decides on therapy and pain medication, plus a physical exam costing $300, leaving her an account balance of $500 plus $50 in interest at the end of the year.

In her second year in Medicare, Ms. Brown remains in the same plan and has her account replenished by $1,700. This sum is added to the $550 carried over from the previous year. Despite the risk, she decides to try to increase her balance by investing in the stock fund. Alas, stock prices tumble by 40 percent, as they did in the early 2000s. Her balance drops to $1,350. Her back pain returns. Now physical therapy is not a medical option. Her account will cover the cost of the injection plus her annual physical but not the surgery her doctor now urgently recommends. She opts for the injection, which is all she can afford, and hopes for the best.

These examples illustrate two important aspects of a consumer-directed system. First, the medical choices that all patients will face—and should face according to advocates of this approach—will be more powerfully influenced by financial considerations than under social insurance or premium support. Second, personal responsibility comes with personal consequences in terms of health, access, quality, and costs. Neither insurers nor the government would offer a safety net for poor choices.

## The Devilish Details

Like all Medicare reforms, consumer-directed health care rests on distinct design choices. Some of the choices are fundamental to the approach itself—that there will be a high deductible, for example. Others can vary and will influence how well the system meets program goals and how acceptable it is to the public, beneficiaries, providers, and policymakers.

### How Is the Deductible Set and What Counts toward It?

Though central to the consumer-directed approach, the high deductible is likely to generate controversy over the level at which it is set. Early efforts to promote MSAs failed, some say, because the deductibles were so high that they discouraged plans from participating and individuals from enrolling. The $2,000 minimum deductible in the Medicare demonstration is less than one-fourth of the maximum deductible in the standard MSAs allowed under Medicare Advantage, an apparent effort to make the option more appealing. On the other hand, a deductible of about $2,000 may be too low to have much effect on consumer behavior. In fact, a $2,000 deductible combined with low out-of-pocket spending limits would result in less cost sharing for certain beneficiaries than now occurs under Medicare. As shown in chapter 2, co-payments for patients with lengthy hospitalizations can vastly exceed any of the stop-loss limits proposed for high-deductible insurance.

It is equally important to determine what spending counts toward the deductible and stop-loss ceilings. In some of today's high-deductible plans, only spending on services or providers covered in the plan network would count. Under a more inclusive standard, any spending on health care would count. For example, drugs not included in the formularies of insurance plans could count toward deductibles and limits on out-of-pocket spending. The more that is counted, the sooner that deductibles and spending limits are reached and insurance coverage begins—and the more costly the plan. The tighter the definition of what counts toward deductibles and stop-loss limits, the greater the financial pressure on enrollees to economize on care and the greater the risk of cost exposure beyond the so-called out-of-pocket maximum. These policy choices directly affect plan costs, demand for care, and, possibly, health outcomes.

To illustrate, research shows a complicated relationship between cost sharing, other insurance limits, and overall costs. One study found that caps on drug benefits reduced patient adherence to drug regimens and increased costs for emergency room visits and nondiscretionary hospitalization. The cost of these unintended effects fully offset reductions in payments for drugs.[37] Another study found that limiting Medicaid recipients to three prescriptions a month saved money on drugs but generated offsetting expenses of other kinds. In the case of schizophrenic patients, the increased costs were seventeen times the savings.[38] Still another study found that the added cost of making ACE inhibitors, a drug used to treat high blood pressure, available free of charge to elderly diabetics saved more than added drug costs by reducing other treatment costs.[39] Paying those with tuberculosis to come to a clinic to be observed swallowing their medications reduced overall spending.[40]

These examples raise several questions. What services, if any, should be excluded from deductibles? When do short-term savings persist, and when do they lead to larger outlays later on? What rules, if any, should govern cost sharing for exempted services? Should all plans have to abide by them? How would separate deductibles and cost sharing be administered? Any refinement of high-deductible coverage could improve efficiency and quality but might increase complexity and government "interference" in a market-oriented model—and reduce consumer direction.

## How Should Personal Accounts Be Funded and Managed?

Setting the size of the personal account is an even more important issue than choosing the deductible. The larger the gap between the personal account deposit and the deductible, the lower the overall cost to the government—but the greater the risk that Medicare enrollees might suffer financial hardship or reduced access to care. Three factors would affect the size of the account: how much Medicare and individuals can contribute to it, how its balances can be invested, and how it can be used.

The consumer-directed Medicare described in this chapter would subsidize individual accounts. Medicare would set a payment for each beneficiary. If an insurer sets its beneficiary deductible high or effectively holds down its own costs, then its bid in relation to the Medicare payment would be low, leaving more left over to deposit in personal accounts. The Medicare account subsidy would then vary in accordance with the insurers' offering and beneficiaries' choices. Accounts would also be affected by the wide variation in per capita health care spending from state to state and from county to county within states. If Medicare fails to take local spending into account, deposits in individual accounts that are linked to identical policies would vary geographically. This payment policy would create concerns about fairness, as the real purchasing power of the accounts would be greater in low-cost areas. To reduce such variations, Medicare could adjust payments to reflect local health cost differences, as it does in the current MSA demonstration. However, experience with Medicare to date has shown that such adjustments are hard to achieve in practice.

Advocates of this approach consider the differentiation in the Medicare contribution to the account an advantage. It allows enrollees to choose the level of risk and amount of the contribution as well as the type and source of health care services. Alternatively, Medicare could set both the deductible and account contribution and require plans to compete on other aspects of the insurance coverage. Fixed deductibles and contributions would simplify

the system and give Medicare rather than insurers control over these critical parameters. However, it would raise questions about fairness because a
fixed contribution would cover varying fractions of health costs, depending
on where the beneficiary lived.

A related question concerns how much beneficiaries themselves should
be permitted to contribute to these tax-favored personal accounts. As with
health savings accounts, the contributions, investment income, and withdrawals would be exempt from taxes. For Medicare enrollees with no tax
liability—who constitute approximately half of all seniors—the value of
these tax advantages is negligible.[41] For upper-income Medicare beneficiaries, however, their worth is considerable. Some limit on the annual contribution to the accounts would be necessary to limit their use as tax
shelters. The current Medicare demonstration caps beneficiary deposits at
$500 less than the deductible.[42] Some policymakers have sought legislation
to allow even greater individual contributions, which would expand the
potential for tax avoidance on commensurately greater investment
income.[43]

Policymakers would also have to establish rules for the investment of personal account balances and for the disposition of unspent funds. The current Medicare demonstration has no restrictions so long as the banks
managing the accounts are legitimate. Expected yields increase with asset
risk. While some beneficiaries would invest their accounts wisely, others
would suffer losses that undermine the program's objective of ensuring
financial access to health care. Regulatory limits on the menu of approved
investments would therefore be essential. In addition, it would be necessary
to decide whether withdrawals for purposes other than paying for health
care would be allowed and, if so, under what circumstances. What would
be the tax penalty for non-health uses? Could unspent balances be transferred to heirs upon death? Would any taxes be imposed on such unspent
balances? These issues are similar to those that have vexed supporters of
individual retirement accounts as an alternative to Social Security.[44]

The answers to these questions would affect attitudes toward personal
accounts. The more that beneficiaries consider accounts to be "their
money," the more likely they are to be cost-conscious in their use of health
care services. If funds could not be used for purposes other than health care
and could not be transferred to heirs at death, account holders might feel
that they have to "use it [for health care] or lose it." On the other hand, if
the funds could be easily withdrawn without penalty, enrollees might be
tempted either to cash out the funds prematurely or to cut back on other

savings and might find themselves financially burdened when serious and protracted illness does occur.

### Will High-Deductible Plans Participate?

Recent experience with the Medicare drug program suggests that insurers would flock to offer coverage in a Medicare market that limits their risk exposure and blocks out a government-run, default plan. However, high-deductible health insurance would carry greater risks for insurers than the drug plans impose. Because high-deductible plans would disproportionately insure the highly variable, very expensive episodes of care, possible losses would be far greater than they are under the drug plan. Hence risk-adjusted payments from Medicare or protection against outlier cases to such plans would be far more important than under the drug plan. If consumer-directed reforms did not include such protections (described in chapter 5), insurers might hesitate to enter the market.

To make sure that high-deductible insurance is available, some have suggested the federal government act as the high-deductible insurer.[45] Medicare could use its existing systems to pay most of the costs that exceed the deductible. It could lift its prohibition on "balance billing" and remove restrictions on private contracting to promote price competition among providers. As the sole plan in the system, it could make personal account contributions uniform and avoid selling costs. Cost would be contained through competition on outlays up to the deductible, not through private insurers' management of costs above the deductible. To purists, however, a Medicare fee-for-service payment system seems inconsistent with the principle of restricted government involvement.[46]

### How to Balance Cost Consciousness and Choice

Experience with Medigap insurance has shown that some seniors are so determined to avoid any outlays when sick that they will buy Medigap coverage even when its premiums exceed the spending that it obviates. Limiting such insurance would raise a difficult question. Why should the government prohibit people from willingly spending their own money for a product sellers are prepared to supply? If every beneficiary has to pay a minimum deductible, is that not contrary to the idea of consumer choice?

The simplest solution, proposed here, would be to permit supplemental coverage but only if it covers part of the deductible and is sold by the same company that offers the basic high-deductible plan. The added premium would have to cover enrollees' increased usage and reduced price sensitivity from decreased cost exposure. An alternative way to keep supplemental insurance while preserving economic incentives would be to tax the added coverage: the more generous it is, the higher the tax. Although such a charge would be difficult to design and politically contentious, it would ensure that supplemental insurance does not undermine the cost-containment goal of consumer-directed insurance reform.

## Assessment

Consumer-directed Medicare is more difficult to assess than social insurance or premium support because there has been less experience with this model. Nevertheless, it has generated much analysis and speculation.

### Ensuring Access

To reiterate, a central goal of Medicare is to promote access to needed health care. The extent to which this goal is achieved under consumer-directed Medicare would depend on both beneficiary behavior and luck. The key to financing care would be to ensure that personal accounts maintain a sufficient balance to cover charges beneficiaries face. Account balances would depend on beneficiaries' choices of plans, investment options, use of health care, and non–health care use of those balances. For beneficiaries who spend little on health care, the account would cover all outlays, essential or discretionary. The same would hold true for high-spending beneficiaries whose previous expenses had remained low long enough for them to build up sizable account balances. However, large gaps could develop between personal account balances and the deductible. Some might prefer plans with low premiums that make small deposits to personal accounts. Some might experience poor investment outcomes. And some will doubtless run into unexpected or persistently high expenses that will drain their accounts.

Access under high-deductible insurance will depend on whether consumers focus on cost by selectively and accurately forgoing low-benefit care while continuing to use needed care. More probably, however, the system would discourage the use of both essential and nonessential services. Although the study sample of the famous RAND Health Insurance Experiment (HIE) excluded seniors and people with disabilities, that behavior is actually what the experimenters observed, resulting in perceptibly adverse effects on the health of poor, but not of non-poor, subjects.[47] More recent evidence suggests that Medicare beneficiaries are more likely than other people to forgo both needed and unneeded care. A study of retirees in California showed that when confronted with increased co-payments for drugs, retirees curtailed use of drugs that controlled acute life-threatening and chronic conditions, as well as those that improved the quality of life. Furthermore, the price sensitivity of medical care utilization among the retirees was greater than that reported in the RAND HIE for the nonelderly.[48]

Further evidence from experience of the nonelderly suggests that access to care under high-deductible plans linked to health savings accounts is worse than it is under comprehensive plans. In one survey, 28 percent of privately insured adults in plans with deductibles less than $1,000 versus 38 percent with deductibles of $1,000 or more and a tax-favored account reported difficulty with access, including the inability to fill a prescription or skipping doses to make a medication last longer.[49] Nearly one-third of those in high-deducible plans—twice the proportion in more comprehensive plans—had delayed or avoided getting health care when sick because of the cost.[50] Financial hardship is also more frequent in consumer-directed health plans than under comprehensive coverage. In another survey, 41 percent of privately insured adults with deductibles of $1,000 or more, versus 23 percent with deductibles of less than $500, reported problems paying medical bills or had accumulated medical debt.[51] Although these results cannot simply be extrapolated to the consumer-directed Medicare proposal outlined here, they do point to the risk of unintended consequences.

Yet another access issue relates to having a local choice of providers. Currently, most physicians and virtually all hospitals accept some or all Medicare patients. On the face of it, consumer-directed Medicare would sustain such access. Unlike network plans, insurers would have little incentive to exclude providers. Even more providers might participate, as they would not have to bother with Medicare's blunt rules and reimbursement methods.[52] On the other hand, physicians would be able to set any fee they liked, and unless individuals and insurance plans were willing to pay those fees, a hierarchy of providers would emerge in which high-price providers would be accessible only to those beneficiaries able to pay. Payments from personal accounts would be entirely the patient's responsibility. In other words, consumer-directed Medicare could unravel the one-tier health system that Medicare helped to create for seniors and people with disabilities.

## Promoting Quality and Satisfaction

Consumer-directed Medicare could improve the quality of care in several ways. Demand for information on quality would almost certainly increase. Beneficiaries would need easy access to useful information on available insurance to determine whether, where, and how much to spend on health care. Experience suggests that the reporting of quality measures, irrespective of how the information is used, improves provider performance.[53] Satisfaction might increase for those who feel constrained by Medicare- or insurance-determined benefit packages. For example, home-bound patients whose required services are not currently covered by Medicare could use their personal accounts to pay for those services. Increased personal involvement in managing medical benefits might improve consumer satisfaction. The choice of physicians would also likely be greater than under premium support—although quite possibly less than it is under Medicare. Experience with managed care during the 1990s suggests that the option to change insurers and providers when perceived quality is low helps improve quality.[54]

However, the proportion of enrollees dissatisfied with consumer-directed health care has been high to date. In a 2007 survey, only 47 percent of those in consumer-directed health plans reported being "extremely" or "very" satisfied compared with 64 percent in traditional plans. Also, more than two-fifths of the enrollees were not satisfied with out-of-pocket costs.[55] Furthermore, those who voluntarily set up a health savings account are not a random sample of the population. Although the Government Accountability Office has found HSA enrollees to be generally satisfied, most of those polled had chosen the HSA from a list of options, so it was not the only plan available. Respondents in one focus group reported that they were unlikely to recommend health savings accounts to those who "use maintenance medication, have a chronic condition, have children, or may not have the funds to meet the high deductible."[56]

A central question for the redesign of Medicare is whether the pressure of health care consumers, competition among private health plans, or regulation through Medicare is most likely to improve program performance. Proponents of consumer-directed health care argue that giving individuals an enlarged financial stake would make them demand—and get—improved outcomes from providers. Critics worry that sick patients, driven by uncertainty and fear, would be incapable of soberly pressuring providers for the best care per dollar of outlay. They suspect that some providers would focus on amenities and on readily visible services, such as high-tech intervention, but would neglect less obvious services, such as hospital practices that minimize infection rates.

## *Controlling Costs*

The consumer-directed model is designed to make federal spending on Medicare predictable. Initial spending would be capped, and in each successive year it would be pegged to a standard index such as per capita income or health expenditures. Consumer-directed Medicare would lower federal spending but it would also lower overall spending if it caused a reduction in prices or use. Research indicates that account holders show heightened price awareness and engage in more price shopping than do other health care purchasers. One survey found that 60 percent of people in high-deductible health plans versus 50 percent in more comprehensive plans checked whether their plans would cover services before seeking care. Similarly, 27 percent of enrollees in high-deductible plans versus 21 percent in more comprehensive plans checked the price of services before getting care.[57] Longer-term savings would be even greater if medical research were redirected to a search for technologies that reduce cost as well as enhance quality. On the other hand, it is unclear whether high-deductible plans and HSAs induced price-sensitive behavior in those who bought into them or enrollees were simply price-sensitive people to begin with. Nor is it clear whether people with chronic illness, mental illness, or long-term care needs—who form a sizable fraction of the Medicare population—will be as cost sensitive as those who have voluntarily enrolled in high-deductible plans.

A system that exposes consumers to increased deductibles would likely reduce use. That was the finding of the RAND HIE. More recent research focusing on retirees (whom the HIE omitted) found that modest increases in cost sharing for physician visits and for prescription drugs significantly lowered use of these two forms of care, but caused partially offsetting increases in expenditures for hospital use.[58] To avoid perverse effects, most high-deductible plans provide first-dollar coverage of preventative care.[59] Best practice for managing chronic disease calls for little or no cost sharing on maintenance drugs and physician visits.[60]

Cost may be difficult to contain for another reason. Most outlays occur during episodes of care that cost far more than any plausible deductible.[61] In 2001, 96 percent of total Medicare spending was incurred by beneficiaries whose spending exceeded $1,340—which equals about $2,000 in 2008, the size of Ms. Brown's deductible if adjusted for medical inflation.[62] Higher deductibles would prevent some episodes of care from reaching the deductible, but once outlays exceed the deductible, high-deductible insurance does little to lower use through price sensitivity. In fact, high-deductible insurance may reduce price sensitivity because once the deductible has been met, cost sharing is lower than in many standard insurance policies and Medicare.[63]

Higher administrative costs under high-deductible plans would offset at least part of any savings from other sources. Medicare's current administrative costs run at about 3–5 percent of outlays.[64] Administration accounts for about 10–15 percent of private large group insurance premiums and 15–30 percent of private individual health insurance premiums.[65] These costs would probably decline in the framework of high-deductible insurance serving all Medicare enrollees, but they would remain far above the program's current administrative costs. People would face additional administrative costs for the management of balances in their personal savings accounts and payments made from them. After enactment of the law creating health savings accounts in 2003, one industry report stated, "over the next five years, financial institutions have the potential to capture $3.5 billion in revenues driven by account and asset manager fees. Health payment processors stand to earn $2.3 billion in processing fees over the same period."[66] These direct costs, and their indirect effect on utilization, would offset at least part of any savings resulting from consumer-directed Medicare.

## Conclusion

Consumer-directed health care, the newest approach for reforming Medicare, fuses libertarian principles and standard economic theory to justify a scaled-back insurance system. It would end coverage of modest outlays that beneficiaries can make themselves. Beneficiaries would be given the resources and responsibility to become wise consumers of care and an effective force for lowering prices and raising quality. Providers would be paid by beneficiaries and high-deductible health plans, not by Medicare. They would have greater incentive to hold down prices and squeeze out medical waste and inefficiency in order to attract new customers and hold old ones. Medicare's outlays would rise less rapidly than under current law. And consumer-directed Medicare would give individuals more control over their health benefits than they would enjoy under other reform models.

Ultimately, the prospects for consumer-directed Medicare rise or fall on the acceptability of its premise—that health care is much like other consumer goods, in the sense that it is best allocated according to the demands of individuals operating in relatively unregulated markets. If people have improved information and a heightened stake in using it, say system advocates, efficiency and quality will improve. To put this premise into practice, consumer-directed Medicare would ask health insurers to pursue their original mission, which is to protect against financial catastrophes rather than manage care. And it would replace Medicare's defined-benefit approach with a defined contribution. Medicare would be a payer, not an insurer.

Whether a consumer-directed system would work as promised and meet Medicare's goals and whether it would save money—not just immediately, but over the long run—is unknown. Increased deductibles would lower use and might hold down prices. They could encourage cost-reducing technological innovation. Financial risk might lead people to take better care of themselves than they do now. On the other hand, selling and other administrative costs would rise. High deductibles would increase the short-term financial costs of adhering to drug regimens, especially when overt symptoms are not present, as is often the case with drugs used to control cholesterol or blood sugar. And seriously ill patients are poorly positioned to influence and evaluate costly interventions.[67] The demand for information to make such assessments would surely increase, but gaps in information would persist for a long time. Inadequate financial protections for people with low income, complicated health needs, low education, or cognitive impairments could jeopardize their access to care.[68]

The political viability of converting Medicare to high-deductible insurance is also in doubt. It would entail an enormous change from the status quo. Deductibles would be significantly higher. The revenue stream to providers from Medicare would dry up. Direct-to-consumer advertising would explode. Moreover, consumer-directed health insurance lacks bipartisan support. Liberals charge that consumer-directed health care would turn Medicare into nothing more than a funding source for an entirely market-run, individually based payment system. That, counter its advocates, is precisely their goal. But the more serious charge is that it could subject enrollees to untenable financial risks and benefit Wall Street more than Main Street. Despite these criticisms, the consumer-directed concept has gained considerable political traction. In chapter 7, we evaluate its proponents' claims alongside those in support of other approaches to Medicare reform.

# 7 | Assessing Medicare Reform Options and Prospects

Almost everyone agrees that Medicare needs to be improved, but not on how to do it.[1] Assessments of what is right and wrong with the program are numerous and conflicting. Some argue that the program is too comprehensive, others that it is not comprehensive enough. Some suggest it pays too much for health care, others too little.

Despite these differences, most reform plans are variations on the three approaches described in chapters 4, 5, and 6. The first, updated social insurance, would allow Medicare to determine benefits and payment rates. The second, premium support, would give each beneficiary a fixed amount to buy private coverage from insurers that would set benefits and provider payments. Consumer-directed Medicare, the third option, would have beneficiaries pay for care from government-supported savings accounts or out of pocket up to a high deductible, after which catastrophic insurance coverage would begin. These approaches mirror those contemplated for the reform of the entire health system.

## Performance of the Current System

Medicare's central objectives are to ensure affordable access to high-quality health care and at the same time control overall

115

costs. These goals are elusive and in mutual conflict. As explained in chapter 3, Medicare does a good job of providing access to covered services. Cost sharing is modest for many services and zero for some, but potentially ruinous for those who suffer protracted hospitalizations. Coverage of some services—mental health, long-term care, and periodic physical examinations—is severely limited. However, Medicare opens the doors to virtually all health care providers in the United States. It also sustains hospitals and other providers in thinly settled areas.

Medicare is unquestionably popular.[2] Its beneficiaries express satisfaction with their coverage far more than do people covered by any other type of health insurance. However, Medicare has been barred from using its market power to improve the quality of care. Congress requires it to reimburse any provider with a license who serves enrollees. Medicare is therefore prohibited from forcing low-quality providers to either improve their skills or drop out of the program. Because Congress has prohibited Medicare from "interfering with the practice of medicine," it has seldom withheld or withdrawn reimbursements for untried or ineffective procedures, or tried to induce physicians and hospitals to increase their practice of cost-effective care, or penalize them for not doing so.

Some of Medicare's quality shortcomings are endemic to the U.S. health system. Cost and use vary widely from place to place without corresponding differences in health outcomes. Most insurers pay for specific services rather than full episodes of care or outcomes. Optimal treatment of seriously ill patients—especially those with multiple conditions who account for the majority of health care spending—requires the cooperation of many practitioners, including physicians, nurses, and technicians.[3] Case histories and test results must also be readily available. Well-managed integrated medical practices promote cooperation among physicians within hospitals and between providers of inpatient and outpatient care. Yet neither Medicare nor private insurers have effectively promoted such cooperative delivery of care.

After a rocky start, Medicare has done about as well—or poorly—as private insurers in controlling per capita spending. Initially, the program contributed to a sharp rise in the price of all health care by covering all incurred hospital costs and paying physicians in a way that spurred fee inflation. By enabling its beneficiaries to access high-cost treatments that were previously unaffordable, it may have underwritten the cost-increasing technological revolution that has reshaped modern medical care.[4] Later,

Medicare's prospective payment systems limited the direct incentives to charge excessive fees. Some analysts attribute the sharp reduction in the duration of hospital stays to Medicare's inpatient prospective payment system.[5] By limiting prices for physician and other services, Medicare has tried to hold down the unit cost of these services as well. Indeed, Medicare has been a leader in efforts to limit the growth of health care spending. All the same, these efforts have not narrowed the margin by which health care spending outpaces income growth. Some of this margin results from a payment and coverage system that does little to discourage low-benefit care. Some occurs because Medicare, like private insurance, pays for cost-increasing technologies. Furthermore, Medicare's payment systems are difficult to update, refine, and replace.

## Summaries of Reform Strategies

Of the three general approaches, social insurance would use Medicare's leverage to improve its performance. This strategy, described in chapter 4, retains the core principle that all beneficiaries are entitled to the same, defined benefits. Medicare's multiple parts would be consolidated in a single system with one premium. In determining payment and benefit policy, Medicare would be given wide authority to modify and overhaul systems to keep the program up to date. It would also be given a stronger mandate to use tools known to improve quality. These changes rest on the assumption that a publicly managed, single payer can do a better job than private insurers or individuals in ensuring access, raising quality, and containing the growth of spending.

Premium support derives from the belief that competition among private plans can slow the growth of total spending by holding down prices and use and can improve quality without unduly restricting access to health care. As described in chapter 5, this approach would replace traditional Medicare with a subsidy that recipients could use to buy private health insurance in a regulated market. Benefit standards, risk adjustment, and oversight would be used to limit risk selection. Beneficiaries could spend their own money to buy more coverage or more choice among providers than the basic subsidy would afford. Insurers would compete for enrollees by providing high-quality services, packaging appealing mixes of benefits, and controlling the growth of premiums. The goal of this competition would be to offer cost-effective care at an affordable price.

Table 7-1. *Comparison of Three Approaches to Medicare Reform*

| Feature | Type of approach | | |
| --- | --- | --- | --- |
| | *Social insurance* | *Premium support* | *Consumer direction* |
| Organizing principle of proposal | Pooled purchasing power and shared risk. | Private plan competition to attract enrollees and lower costs. | Individual control and liability for health care dollars. |
| Who determines benefits and cost sharing? | Medicare determines services covered and cost sharing; Expert panels determine coverage based on cost-effectiveness standards. | Private plans determine benefits and cost sharing within legislated parameters. | Individuals determine services purchased with tax-favored personal savings accounts; High-deductible plans provide catastrophic coverage within legislated parameters. |
| How are payments to plans, providers, or both determined? | Government pays providers directly; Rates negotiated or set service by service and based on performance; Competitive bidding for some services. | Private plans are paid a fixed (risk-adjusted) fee per beneficiary by Medicare based on bids; Plans compete for customers on the basis of service, price, and quality; Capitation creates pressure on insurance plans to negotiate low rates from providers. | Medicare pays for high-deductible insurance; Medicare makes an annual deposit to individual accounts, risk-adjusted at plan level; Individuals, using premium, price, and quality information, shop for the lowest-price, highest-quality care that best meets their needs. |

| | | | |
|---|---|---|---|
| Which providers are covered? | Enrollees may use any qualified provider; Financial incentives encourage use of high-quality, low-cost providers. | Private plans determine provider networks within government-set limits; Allow out-of-network use with higher cost sharing; Capitation creates pressure to exclude high-cost providers. | Individuals may use any provider; Providers may turn away patients. |
| How is quality encouraged? | Medicare develops quality systems to determine participating providers; Extra pay for high-quality providers; Financial incentives (for example, lower cost sharing) for enrollees to use high-quality providers. | Private plans seek to improve quality to encourage enrollment. | Individuals receive information on quality of providers; Approach relies on choice and change of provider to promote quality of care. |

Consumer-directed Medicare would deputize individuals, supported by improved information and goaded by economic incentives, to shop for medical services at the price and quality they desire. Medicare's financial responsibility for paying for health care would be limited to subsidizing high-deductible plans and making deposits into beneficiaries' tax-favored, personal savings accounts that would be available to pay for health care. Unspent balances would roll over from year to year. No backup funding from Medicare would be available for those who exhaust their accounts. High-deductible plans would compete for beneficiaries as they do under premium support, although with little oversight from Medicare. The task of monitoring quality would fall to beneficiaries.

These three approaches differ in principle and in operation (see table 7-1). Benefits and cost sharing are determined collectively under a social insurance model, by private plans reflecting consumer preferences under premium support, and by enrollees themselves under consumer-directed Medicare. The determination of what providers get paid is centralized under social insurance, delegated to private plans under premium support, and left to providers and beneficiaries under consumer-directed Medicare. Free choice of provider would remain a key feature of Medicare as a social insurer, although administrators might exercise their new authority to either discourage the use of or exclude low-quality providers. Under premium support, the choice of providers would depend on the breadth of the provider network in the particular plan the enrollee joins. Consumer-directed Medicare would provide beneficiaries with information on prices and quality of providers, but they could receive care from any provider who would see them and whose services they could afford. Under both premium support and consumer-directed Medicare, quality improvement would depend largely on whether insurers see quality promotion as a good marketing device, while it would be built into the functions of a reformed social insurance program. The government could support research to identify cost-effective treatments under all three reform options.

All three options would have a wide impact beyond Medicare—on people, providers, and the health system at large. For example, increased cost sharing would have implications for Social Security and the retirement security of some seniors. Raising Medicare quality standards would have systemwide effects since the same providers that treat beneficiaries care for other Americans. And reductions in Medicare coverage would likely cause uncompensated care to increase, thereby boosting charges on others in the complicated, multipayer U.S. health system.

Table 7-2. *Ranking of Approaches to Medicare Reform*

| Medicare objective | | Social insurance | Premium support | Consumer direction |
|---|---|---|---|---|
| Ensuring access | Financial | High | Medium | Low |
| | Physical | High | Low | Medium |
| Promoting quality | Optimal care | Medium | Medium | Low |
| | Satisfaction | High | Medium | Low |
| Controlling costs | Total | Low | High | Medium |
| | Government | Low | Medium | High |

## How Do the Reform Options "Stack Up"?

Our rankings of the three reform options reflect the findings of health services research, predictions about how plans would behave, and our own values. Other rankings may be defensible as well. Our purpose is to encourage readers to understand Medicare's goals, to recognize the tradeoffs among these goals, and to form their own opinions.

### Comparisons in Summary

Given the complexity of Medicare and the tradeoffs among its goals, no reform strategy seems best in all dimensions (see table 7-2). The social insurance approach would do the best job of preserving and improving access and satisfaction. It has done well historically, and a reformed version might do somewhat better. It may improve performance in controlling total and government spending but to a lesser degree than alternatives. If Medicare's administrators were empowered to use its market leverage aggressively, the program could spearhead a revolution in the quality of care.

Premium support would likely do the best job of controlling the growth of total health care spending on the Medicare population. Aggressive management of care by insurers could advance quality. But such cost-control tools as limited networks of providers and use management would lower satisfaction, physical access to care, and possibly financial access to care if risk selection persists.

Consumer-directed Medicare is most likely to control federal spending but otherwise offers the least promise of advancing Medicare's other goals. It could reduce access to care, especially among those with high need. Despite its name, it is likely to lower enrollee satisfaction. And it is not clear that patients are well positioned to demand high-quality care.

### Promoting Access

Access to health services encompasses both affordability and proximity. Health insurance should cover enough of the cost of services to permit appropriate use. The plan's payment and system design should support adequate geographic availability. Medicare performs well on both scores for covered services but still suffers important gaps in coverage. The payment system should also signal value, discouraging frivolous use and encouraging cost-effective use of services such as those for prevention or drugs for chronic disease. On this score, Medicare's current performance is decidedly mixed.

SOCIAL INSURANCE. The social insurance approach would not only sustain but also enhance access. A revamped social insurance program would rationalize premiums and cost sharing and could integrate assistance for low-income beneficiaries into the core program. Although its payment and quality systems would change, providers would likely continue to participate in Medicare at high rates throughout the country. These changes would simplify the program for patients and for providers alike. Social insurance gives no explicit economic incentive to limit use. Providers are paid more to do more, and beneficiaries face no cap on physician services and other forms of care. Such open-ended coverage has led to overuse but puts beneficiaries at least risk of forgoing needed care. However, a single insurance plan is not likely to be optimal for everyone, as not all beneficiaries are "average." A uniform benefit design will poorly serve some beneficiaries in need of specialized services, such as those with mental illness. Even allowing for such gaps, Medicare as a social insurance program would continue to rank high in ensuring financial and physical access to care under the reforms described here.

PREMIUM SUPPORT. Premium support is designed to ensure access to needed health care. It incorporates guaranteed issue and pure community rating of premiums. These standards are stronger than those in most U.S. health insurance markets. Risk adjustment, limits on benefit variation, reinsurance, and rules regarding network adequacy would curb discrimination against sick and costly beneficiaries.

Premium support is also designed to encourage insurers to limit use. Plans would be paid a flat sum per beneficiary. To be competitive on cost, they would have to control the prices paid for various services used by enrollees. It may be easier and more profitable to lower the use of high-cost services than to extract price discounts, especially in areas with little provider competition. Indeed, lowering the use of relatively low-benefit, high-cost services is a goal of premium support. The challenge is how to do so without also denying care that is needed or strongly desired. If the system fails to differentiate between essential and inessential care, it runs the risk of provoking a public and political backlash, as occurred toward managed care during the 1990s. The incentive to limit use, with the attendant risk of reduced access, is inherent in premium support.

Flexibility of benefit design, a key attribute of premium support, can also reduce access. Ideally, beneficiaries would be fully informed about coverage, cost sharing, and premiums and would choose the plan that best meets their perceived needs. This ideal, alas, is seldom realized. Health insurance is complex. Even if benefit packages are limited to a few prototypes, many enrollees will not fully understand them. In addition, beneficiaries' wants regarding health benefits are uncertain and changeable. Benefit design can also be used for risk selection. Whether currently available risk-adjustment formulas or others that may be devised in the near future will eliminate enough of the profit from enrolling low-cost patients remains unclear.[6] If they do not, plans could discourage high-cost beneficiaries from enrolling by limiting coverage or by raising cost sharing on services they seek.

Premium support would likely reduce access to at least some providers. Private plans tend to limit rosters of approved providers as an important management tool. Plans hold down prices and influence practice patterns by forming physician networks, selecting hospitals, and structuring payments to them. In addition, some use cost-saving devices, such as requiring enrollees to see "gatekeepers" before making appointments with specialists. Under premium support, insurers could offer fee-for-service plans with unfettered access to "any willing provider," but enrollees would have to be willing and able to pay for them. The tradeoff between free access to providers and effective cost control illustrates the inescapable conflict among the legitimate objectives of Medicare reform.

CONSUMER-DIRECTED MEDICARE. By definition, a budget-neutral, consumer-directed Medicare would provide the same total financial support for beneficiaries as the other models, but it would be structured differently. The strength of the high-deductible approach—its emphasis on cost-sensitive demand for care by patients—is also a potential weakness. The same cost sensitivity that limits demand for genuinely low-value care would also limit demand for care that patients erroneously undervalue, such as maintenance and preventive therapies. This problem could be ameliorated by excluding high-benefit services from deductibles, but doing so encroaches on the model's premise that consumers know best. Access to care would also depend on account balances. High use would deplete account balances. Beneficiaries with high but legitimate health care needs would therefore be at greater risk of having inadequate Medicare assistance to pay for them. Increased deductibles would have little effect on demand for such urgent services as hospitalization after a heart attack or cancer chemotherapy, but they would change the distribution of out-of-pocket spending. The bottom line is that access to care would depend on the ability of beneficiaries to choose plans wisely, to invest their account balances prudently, and to use care sensibly—and, most important, it would depend on the state of their health.

Physical access to providers is also important. Consumer-directed health insurance would not impose explicit limits on which providers beneficiaries could see. At the same time, providers would no longer be paid according to Medicare's fee schedule and could charge whatever the market would bear. Unless their personal accounts had grown, low-income beneficiaries would be unable to afford high-priced providers, who now serve all Medicare patients irrespective of income. Unless current subsidies to rural providers were retained, access to care in rural areas would dwindle. Hence, consumer-directed Medicare might reduce access to providers in ways that are less transparent than the explicit networks created by health plans under premium support.

### Improving Quality

Which reform would do the best job of promoting high-quality care and beneficiary satisfaction? Whatever model is adopted, the evidence base must be strengthened in order to better define optimal care. Paying for research to build this knowledge base must be a public responsibility, because knowledge, once developed, would be freely available to all. The rapid introduction of information technology would enable physicians, hospitals, and other providers to exchange information as easily as households and businesses now do via e-mail. High-quality care, particularly for patients with multiple illnesses, requires tracking, monitoring, and the coordination and cooperation of multiple providers. It also requires greater focus on prevention and control of chronic conditions. None of the three reform strategies has a clear advantage in furthering these goals. But they offer different tools and incentives to promote quality and would likely affect satisfaction in different ways.

SOCIAL INSURANCE. Medicare has shown that it can "raise the bar" on provider behavior through its rules for program participation. At its inception, the program ended racial segregation in southern hospitals. In recent years, it has promoted access to emergency rooms and language services in hospitals. Medicare could similarly enforce quality standards by setting conditions for participation. It could require hospitals to report quality indicators, reveal medical errors, and institute remedial actions. It could organize regional quality forums that hold local providers accountable for how they practice. It could use rewards and penalties to improve adherence to guidelines. Because few providers can do without Medicare's business, these incentives would be effective.

However, some question whether a public health plan can be as effective as private plans at improving quality. Would regulation or market forces encourage "best practices" most effectively? Medicare's very size and dominance may reduce its ability to refine and implement quality systems. Smaller, private plans would be less subject to political constraints and more nimble than a government bureaucracy in defining, refining, and measuring quality and implementing management measures necessary to improve it. Consumers could improve quality to the extent that information is available and use is discretionary—but neither circumstance exists now for most high-cost or volume services.

When it comes to patient satisfaction, a reformed social insurance program like Medicare excels. Primarily because of its performance in providing access and its reliability, Medicare is currently the most popular form of health insurance. The changes under an improved social insurance program would only enhance these features and its popularity. But these advantages would entail higher spending than do the alternatives.

PREMIUM SUPPORT. Some experts believe that quality improvement would be best achieved through local, coordinated systems of care.[7] High-quality care is most apparent in hospital-based systems or large physician groups that design processes and workflow around best practices. Premium support would shift from paying providers for specific services to paying plans for all care for an enrollee. Private plans could easily embrace integrated health care delivery. They could also compete on quality performance. Private and public purchasers are now using quality report cards to assess managed care plans, although evidence on whether they improve quality remains inconclusive.[8]

Whether plans would in fact compete on quality is uncertain. So is the ultimate market dominance of plans that choose to compete on quality. Some quality improvements that lower spending later increase cost now. Unless potential enrollees are willing to pay more up front for better outcomes down the road or plans are willing to invest in quality improvements whose benefits do not accrue for a long time, much quality improvement will lack market appeal. Furthermore, plans will continue to have a market incentive to gratify enrollees' demands for the latest technology or treatment, even if it is untested or of low value.[9] Plans rated top on quality have not always become dominant in their particular markets.

Consumer satisfaction, one measure of quality, would be difficult to maintain under premium support. Cost-reducing procedures, such as prior authorization, have long been unpopular. High users of care or people who develop health problems after they enroll in a plan are especially likely to resist policies intended to discourage use. Recent overpayments to private plans underscore the tradeoff between cost control and enrollee satisfaction. These bonuses have allowed private plans to offer richer benefits than are available in the traditional Medicare program and to downplay the restrictions on use of care that lower costs—and satisfaction. Healthy seniors have welcomed the benefit flexibility of private plans and feel few of its constraints. Thus satisfaction under premium support would depend on the rate at which Congress sets Medicare payments, as well as on the competitive strategies adopted by insurers.

CONSUMER-DIRECTED MEDICARE. In practice, many beneficiaries would find it difficult to balance cost and quality wisely. Reliable information on quality performance is scarce. Even if such information were plentiful, many Medicare enrollees would have limited ability to use it effectively, especially if they are old and frail, have complex health problems, or are suffering from acute illness or injury.

In some instances, consumer-directed Medicare would surely increase satisfaction. Beneficiaries would be able to use personal accounts to pay for services not covered by Medicare. However, the experience of the nonelderly who have enrolled in consumer-directed health plans has revealed dissatisfaction with plan complexity, out-of-pockets costs, and the time burden to inform themselves about health care cost, quality, and treatment alternatives.[10] These enrollees have expressed less overall satisfaction with their plans as well as their care than the nonelderly enrolled in traditional comprehensive health plans.[11]

### Cost Control

With Medicare spending projected to outpace revenues in the near future, cost control is a key goal of program reform. It would be possible to hold down federal outlays simply by shifting costs to enrollees, but balancing the public budget in this way would undermine Medicare's fundamental purpose. Accordingly, "cost control" must apply not just to what taxpayers spend but also to the total cost of health care used by the Medicare population. Many fail to recognize this distinction and thus overlook two important facts. First, no amount of cost control under any of the reform options will obviate the need for higher taxes if Medicare is to continue making high-quality health care available to the elderly and people with disabilities. Second, the three reforms will not be equally effective in controlling health care spending. The social insurance option will be the least effective in slowing the growth of both total and government spending on the Medicare population unless Congress authorizes far more government regulation of the price and style of health care delivered than it has yet accepted. Higher outlays may mean greater access and the potential for superior quality, but they require larger tax increases than the other options do. The same is true in reverse: lower spending may be achieved by premium support and consumer-directed Medicare, but the "cost" of cost control may be diminished access and less improvement in quality than under a social insurance model. American voters cannot escape these tradeoffs and must consider them if they are to fully understand how the three Medicare reform strategies differ.

SOCIAL INSURANCE. The social insurance strategy would rely primarily on administered prices and Medicare's considerable purchasing leverage to control costs. Eliminating private insurers from the system would increase leverage, reduce complexity, and lower administrative costs. Deductibles and cost sharing would play an important but secondary role in cost control.

Other nations have successfully used government budget control or regulations to limit total health care spending. Since Medicare accounts for about 40 percent of hospital revenues and 25 percent of physician revenues, few hospitals could survive without Medicare's business, nor could many physicians.[12] The fact that many other payers follow Medicare's lead on pricing and coverage means the program has more leverage to limit the amount and growth of total spending than its own market share suggests. If Medicare had more flexibility to adapt and change its payment systems, its leverage would be that much greater.

In addition, the large volume of data available to a social insurance system would facilitate the evaluation of new and existing medical procedures, drugs, and devices to determine whether they deliver sufficient added benefits to justify their increased costs. Other countries, including Great Britain and Australia, have created and supported organizations to carry out such evaluations. Their studies of promised benefits and expected costs have undergirded decisions on whether or not to cover new interventions.

Despite these advantages, the degree to which social insurance could control costs is uncertain. First, setting prices consistently at the "right level" for tens of thousands of hospital diagnoses, physician office services, and various drugs and medical devices is probably impossible.[13] At a technical level, Medicare is not the only payer, and allocating overhead costs is inevitably arbitrary. Second, fee-for-service payment leaves service use uncontrolled. Social insurance does not cap Medicare payments, the key cost control of premium support and consumer-directed insurance. Even if a reformed Medicare used payment policy and cost sharing to discourage low-value care, providers would still profit from supplying more services. As long as the expected benefit is positive, patients who may be desperate for relief or a cure would seek it. Lastly, history suggests that there is little political willingness to use explicit cost controls for health care; those in premium support and consumer-directed Medicare are implicit. These weaknesses would be partly offset by lower administrative costs and the leverage of a large market share. On balance, however, we believe that updated social insurance would have more control over both overall and government costs than the current system but less than would premium support or consumer-directed Medicare.

PREMIUM SUPPORT. Medicare under premium support would control the growth of spending in three ways. First, it would cap per beneficiary Medicare spending by the government. Capitation gives private plans powerful incentives to hold down prices, control use, and curb waste. Second, private plans would have the means as well as the incentive to contain spending growth. Within legislated parameters, they could design benefits, set formularies, create provider networks, and regulate access to new technology. All of these powers would help them provide promised benefits within a fixed government subsidy. Third, plans would have to compete for enrollees. Although such competition might take the form of a technological "arms race," low prices and good value for money will be powerful selling points. Competition for enrollees would also prevent cost-containment strategies from deviating too far from consumers' preferences. A very limited drug formulary, for example, would lower costs but probably deter enrollment as well.

However, some aspects of premium support could erode its savings potential. For one, private plan competition for enrollees would raise marketing and administrative costs. For another, plans might compete by covering high-cost and low-value but popular services. More important, the potential savings of premium support depend on accurate risk adjustment. Insufficient risk adjustment would enable plans to engage in risk selection, which would mean that Medicare would overpay for low-cost beneficiaries, eroding savings from improved efficiency. Nevertheless, of the three models, premium support would probably be the most effective at containing overall costs. The incentives to reduce both price and use are strong.

However, the government share of potential savings may not be commensurate with overall savings. Plans could set their bids to push up the government benchmark and use the added payments to compete for new customers by adding benefits or rebating premiums to enrollees.[14] This has been their preferred way to attract enrollees in recent history. In that event, the same incentives that drive down costs would push up the government share of costs.

CONSUMER-DIRECTED MEDICARE. High-deductible insurance linked to personal accounts would make beneficiaries the principal agents of cost control. The power of high-deductible insurance to reduce service use has been well established by the RAND Health Insurance Experiment and subsequent research.[15] However, overall savings would be offset by other effects. Consumer-directed Medicare would lower average cost sharing for some high-use beneficiaries who face substantial out-of-pocket costs under the current program as they would be completely insured once they passed the stop-loss threshold. Conversely, because cost-minimizing deductibles and coinsurance for such services as preventive care and maintenance drugs are zero or even negative, consumer-directed insurance could boost long-run costs if these services were subject to deductibles. Furthermore, selling costs, advertising, and other administrative costs would be higher than under the current program. And the ability of individuals to drive down physician fees or hospital prices is unproven.

Consumer-directed Medicare would affect total health care spending in complex ways, increasing cost sharing for some patients and lowering it for others. It would also have multiple effects on the federal budget. Personal accounts would shelter some currently taxable capital income, tending to boost deficits. But Congress would directly control the amounts deposited in personal accounts and paid toward high-deductible health insurance premiums. Thus consumer-directed Medicare holds the potential for more *budget* control, if not more *overall* cost control, than the other options do.

## Summary and Tradeoffs

On balance, the expanded social insurance version of Medicare would provide more financial and physical access but would likely save less than the other models. With no per beneficiary cap on spending, it removes the financial incentive to cut back on care—needed or unneeded. Those who use little health care would be clear winners under consumer-directed health care. Their personal accounts would accumulate growing balances that could eventually be used for other purposes. Under premium support, risk adjustment could reduce, but probably not eliminate, the incentive to stint on services that attract high-cost enrollees. Premium support would encourage plans to use provider networks to control costs, thereby limiting choice of providers. An unintended side effect could well be the emergence of a two-tiered system under which people with few means could no longer afford high-cost providers.

In the promotion of high-quality care, each of these three options has important advantages. Social insurance would have access to a huge database for quality measurement. Furthermore, it would implement new rules to improve practice. The government could, and in our view should, support such research regardless of which of the three reform options is chosen. Premium support would increase the use of integrated group plans, a promising mode for delivering high-quality care. Consumer-directed Medicare would rely on individual patients to monitor quality. While advocates of this reform strategy argue that consumers can do this job, we believe that many Medicare beneficiaries fail to understand what elements of health care make for high quality and often cannot exercise a positive influence through the market.

The potential impact of these models on satisfaction is more predictable. Overall satisfaction with Medicare would likely increase under a simpler social insurance system. As with Medicare Advantage, premium support would likely appeal more to healthy than to sick beneficiaries. Experience to date suggests that some people prefer the unbounded and unmanaged choices of consumer-directed health care but that many are dissatisfied by their level of out-of-pocket costs.

Consumer-directed Medicare would give Congress direct control over government spending. Congress would set flat, fixed contributions to personal accounts and the premiums for high-deductible plans. It would have little control over total health care spending by the Medicare population, however, as providers would be free to set any fees the market would bear, while individuals would be left to distinguish between high- and low-value care. Of the three models, premium support would have the greatest potential to reduce overall costs because of its control over both prices and use. At the same time, the bidding behavior of plans could keep government savings down. Although social insurance would control the growth of spending better than the current program does, it would do less in this regard than models with expenditure caps.

Clearly, each strategy has both strengths and weaknesses. Premium support and consumer-directed Medicare would contain spending growth better but provide less access than social insurance. Very sick beneficiaries could face higher cost sharing under premium support or consumer-directed health insurance than under social insurance. The consumer model would prevent seniors with low incomes, poor investment returns, or very large health expenses from building sufficient account balances to give them access to the doctor of their choice. Because it lacks cost caps, social insurance would protect access to care but do less to manage care and costs. Satisfaction among beneficiaries is positively related to spending, which means the more aggressive the cost containment—for example, through tight provider networks or high deductibles—the lower the satisfaction of beneficiaries. But taxpayers would resist the higher taxes that a costly program requires.

Ultimately, the tradeoffs a society tolerates depend on the priorities of its citizens. Some place higher value on ensuring financial access and thus would accept relatively uncontrolled spending and the implied taxes to maintain it. Some believe spending limits are necessary to spare the nation from unaffordable increases in the cost of Medicare and thus might even accept health care rationing. Some would give top priority to consumer autonomy. And some would look first at the potential negatives of a proposal, such as the possible creation of a two-tier or multitier health care system under consumer-directed Medicare. The president and Congress will decide how to balance these values in national law and policy, but the public, providers, and patients will shape those decisions.

## The Politics of Medicare Reform

With so many interests at stake, politics is bound to have a major impact on Medicare policy, as it clearly has in the past. Fiery political controversy surrounded Medicare's enactment, as described in chapter 1. After three decades of relative calm, it resurfaced in the mid-1990s, when the largely bipartisan support for Medicare as a social insurance program began to crumble.[16]

### Social Insurance

Medicare is grounded in values of equity and political solidarity. Like other forms of social insurance, it rests on a tradition that places the common good above individualism—more liberal than conservative, more Democratic than Republican. Medicare relies on regulation more than competition to achieve its goals. Thus it is not a coincidence that the decline of its political popularity coincided with Republican assumption of the control of Congress in 1994. Nor is it surprising that, after gaining control of the White House as well, Republicans proposed far-reaching changes embodied in the Medicare Modernization Act (MMA) of 2003—a drug benefit based on premium support, a premium support demonstration, expanded consumer-directed plan options, and increased payments to private plans in Medicare Advantage.

The Medicare Modernization Act in turn triggered a backlash from supporters of social insurance. As soon as the private insurance model for delivering prescription drugs became a reality, the idea that Medicare should use its buying leverage to negotiate prices for prescription drugs gained momentum, to the chagrin of those favoring a market of competing private prescription drug insurers.[17]

As a social insurance program, Medicare retains the political "home-court advantage." Fear of change is a powerful force in the politics of Medicare, as illustrated by the 1995 budget showdown between President Bill Clinton and the Republican-dominated Congress at the time, led by House Speaker Newt Gingrich. As part of its effort to balance the federal budget, the congressional leadership proposed capping Medicare spending and raising premiums. Through radio addresses, conferences, and analyses, the Clinton administration and Democrats in Congress raised public concern about the changes. Though derided by critics as "Medagoguing," the strategy of reminding seniors of the advantages of the current program helped defeat the proposed Medicare cuts.[18]

Medicare's familiarity as a social insurance program is at once a political strength and a weakness. Beneficiaries may complain about Medicare's peculiarities, but they have come to understand by and large what is and is not covered and how much they must pay for services. Providers often complain about the amount they are paid but rarely about the timeliness, and never about the large share of their income that Medicare payments provide.

Critics of the social insurance model see its uniformity as a weakness, arguing that no single plan can optimally serve all beneficiaries. Many also doubt that a program serving 44 million beneficiaries can be as agile in adapting to new services or in implementing administrative innovations as smaller private plans operating outside the political spotlight. Under the cover of broad rules crafted from afar, they add, providers have found ways to up-code bills and charge for inappropriate services. Critics have also tarred Medicare as "government-run health care," a term of contempt in many quarters. During the 1993–94 health reform debate, for example, plans to increase government regulation and insurance subsidies were said to have "the efficiency of the Post Office with the compassion of the IRS."[19] President George W. Bush, in urging increased funding for private plans in Medicare, asserted that many programs for saving and improving lives and reducing health care costs are not part of Medicare's defined benefits: "Many are only available through Medicare's private plans, and that's important to understand. As we discuss Medicare and its reform, it's important to understand that the defined benefit plan in Medicare limits the capacity of seniors to meet their needs. And that doesn't seem right to me."[20]

Whether concerns about big government resonate with the general public is not clear, especially since Medicare is one of the most popular government programs. Oddly, many beneficiaries do not believe that it is a government program.[21] To them, Medicare looks like private insurance that enables them to see private providers. This formidable base of affection for Medicare as social insurance will continue to shape debate about Medicare reform.

## Premium Support

The political advantages of premium support arise from its philosophical position midway between a "monolithic" social insurance plan and an individual "ownership society" approach to health care delivery that can therefore appropriate some of the appeal of both. Beneficiaries may choose benefits, within bounds, to fit their needs. Private plans can promptly cover the latest drugs or surgeries without exposing beneficiaries to high deductibles. At the same time, premium support does not include the huge array of choices inherent in consumer-directed coverage, offering instead insurance choices with regulatory backstops.

Some aspects of premium support entail political liabilities. Critics see capped funding as a backdoor way to end guaranteed access to health care. With the reliance on private insurers rather than a public program to make key decisions, many fear that "bean counters" or "nameless HMO bureaucrats" will control life-or-death decisions. While political oversight could allay these concerns, it would also threaten the ability of plans to compete and contain costs. This tension helps explain the stiff opposition to premium support. Even with a supportive Republican president and Congress in 2003, premium support advanced only as a demonstration project that does not begin until 2010.

Although it would be harder to win favor for a premium support system than for an updated version of the current system, each new generation of enrollees has more experience with managed care than did its predecessors. Enrollment in Medicare Advantage has risen dramatically since 2004. All beneficiaries in fee-for-service Medicare get their drug benefit through a premium-support system. The result may well be increasing acceptance of premium support.

### Consumer-Directed Medicare

Political conservatives with a libertarian bent remain the chief constituency for consumer-directed Medicare. Its high deductibles and accounts appeal to those who blame a lack of cost consciousness for high U.S. health care spending. Its emphasis on information, price transparency, and unfettered choice of providers and insurers expresses a trust in market solutions. It has given conservatives a substantive and creative idea to present in health policy debates that the political left has tended to dominate. The model's roots in economic theory have also given it an audience among editorial boards and policy "elites."

The appeal of consumer-directed care to the public and Medicare beneficiaries remains untested. To be sure, many of the "young elderly" have managed personal retirement accounts. Many are comfortable looking for information on the Internet. And the ability to use personal savings accounts for services not currently covered by Medicare, such as vision care or personal care services, would attract many. Yet few nonelderly Americans have enrolled in consumer-directed health plans. Those who have done so generally report lower satisfaction than enrollees in traditional plans even though they enrolled voluntarily.[22] Moreover, the argument that Americans are overinsured and that less insurance would reduce spending clashes with the public discontent with high premiums and increased cost sharing. Medicare already covers a smaller proportion of total health care spending by seniors than private insurance covers for the rest of the population.[23] Asking the elderly and people with disabilities to be "at risk" for more will be a hard sell.

For these reasons, consumer-directed Medicare faces the largest political challenges. It could probably be implemented, if at all, only with a long phase-in, which means that its impact on Medicare and on the health care system would be muted and distant.

## Incremental Reform

Large-scale Medicare reform of any stripe will face daunting political challenges. The financial stakes are huge. Medicare spending exceeded $400 billion in 2007—more than nearly all other nations spend in total on health care, and far more than every other U.S. public program except Social Security and national defense.[24] It supports whole industries. The income security of seniors and people with disabilities depends on it. And Medicare is so central a cog in the entire health system that seemingly small changes could produce widespread reverberations. For these reasons, Medicare reform has historically occurred gradually.

Short of comprehensive reform, several steps could be taken to improve Medicare. Some are consistent with all three reform strategies. Social insurance, premium support, and consumer-directed Medicare would all work better with improved information about the efficacy of various medical interventions. Improved information and instruments to transfer that knowledge throughout the delivery system would benefit providers and patients. Similarly, provider quality could be evaluated at the national or regional level, regardless of how Medicare is reformed. New incentives to improve performance or to reward superior performance are possible. Providers could be given information on how their performance compares with that of their peers. Remedial training could be offered to those whose performance is lagging. Payments could be based on performance to a greater extent than is now done. And those who do not meet minimum performance standards could be debarred from the program.

Incremental reform can blend elements of the different models. Traditional Medicare could harness some aspects of market competition. Payments for integrated systems of care, used by private plans in premium support, could be imported into the traditional program. So, too, could competitive contracting for selected services. In addition, increased deductibles and cost sharing could be applied to low-benefit services. Reduced deductibles and cost sharing or none at all—even subsidies—could be tied to underlying health status and used for services likely to lower total spending, such as osteoporosis screening for elderly women. In short, there is no reason why social insurance should forgo the proven incentives to shape behavior in ways that improve outcomes or save money.

Medicare could also benefit from incremental reform of payments to Medicare Advantage plans. Provisions of the MMA boosted payments to such plans excessively. After adjustments for enrollee characteristics, payments are well above those of the traditional program. These overpayments permit Medicare Advantage plans to provide additional benefits beyond those required by Medicare or to reduce premiums. However welcome such benefits or rebates are to enrollees in Medicare Advantage, the overpayments that produce them violate the principle that competition should occur on a level playing field. Moreover, the Medicare actuary reports that their existence pushes the projected date of insolvency of the Hospital Insurance trust fund forward in time by eighteen months.[25]

Some blends of the major approaches to Medicare reform could do more harm than good. For example, one superficially appealing way of introducing consumer-directed Medicare would be to promote it alongside managed care plans and traditional Medicare, with incentives for enrollment. Although allowed under current law, such offerings would be troubling. Differences in benefit designs would encourage beneficiaries with different risk profiles to sort themselves into different plans to a degree that feasible risk adjustment could not offset. Such sorting would raise program costs and jeopardize access.

## The Larger Context for Medicare Reform

Medicare's past and current accomplishments form the backdrop against which reform options should be considered. Medicare has improved access to health care for the elderly and people with disabilities. It has enhanced financial security among the old and frail. It has been both an engine of change in the health system and a source of continuity by sustaining providers in underserved communities. It has created payment standards used by other insurers. It has earned and sustained extraordinary popularity.

Despite these accomplishments, Medicare faces current and future challenges that will force major change. Rising per beneficiary health care spending combined with a rapidly growing beneficiary population promises large expenditure increases, which in turn will require higher taxes or reduced coverage. Meanwhile, many providers complain about low fees, beneficiaries complain about benefit gaps, and Medicare's focus on improving quality remains weak.

Distinct ideas on Medicare reform exist, in the form of the three approaches set forth in this book: social insurance, premium support, and consumer-directed Medicare. Which pure approach one supports depends largely on one's values. Because of the need for political compromise, policymakers will likely draw on all three for incremental reform. We have tried to provide sufficient insight to foster an appreciation of the types of hybrid policies that Congress will consider in the coming years.

It is important to reiterate that none of these options will stop the total cost of Medicare from rising—a lot. The number of beneficiaries is projected to double by 2045.[26] The growth of per beneficiary health care spending is almost certain to continue to exceed the growth of per beneficiary income. These inexorable forces will create an exceedingly difficult environment for reform. Rates of taxes earmarked for Medicare have not been increased for over two decades. Without increased revenue, it will be impossible for Medicare to ensure access to care or to protect the elderly and people with disabilities from the spiraling costs of health care and the ensuing threat to their income and retirement security.

Medicare, though important, accounts for less than a quarter of personal health care spending.[27] Systemic reforms in the U.S. health care system would do far more to control Medicare spending than any reform in the program alone. Policies such as promulgating an evidence-based benefit design, steering patients toward high-value services, and reorienting payment policy toward the prevention of acute and chronic diseases have the potential to curtail spending across the population, not just among the elderly. Systemwide health reform is the best way to make Medicare economically sustainable and enable it to provide beneficiaries with high-quality and affordable health care.

# Payment Systems for Special Hospitals

Long-term care hospitals (LTCHs) provide postacute care for patients with clinically complex, often ventilator-dependent conditions.[1] Inpatient rehabilitation facilities (IRFs) provide intensive inpatient rehabilitation services such as physical, occupational, or speech therapy largely to patients with one or more of thirteen qualifying medical conditions, including stroke, burns, hip fracture, or major joint replacement.[2] Inpatient psychiatric facilities (IPFs) generally furnish short-term acute care to beneficiaries with mental illnesses or alcohol- and drug-related problems.[3]

Overall, these special hospitals depend heavily on Medicare but absorb only 4 percent of Medicare's expenditures.[4] Since January and October 2002, respectively, Medicare has paid IRFs and LTCHs prospective per discharge rates based primarily on patient characteristics (for example, age, sex, and diagnoses), the facility's wage index, and facility characteristics (for example, location and teaching status).[5] In January 2005 Medicare began a three-year transition to a prospective payment system (PPS) for IPFs similar to that for LTCHs and IRFs, the major exception being that IPFs receive case-mix adjusted per diem payments that decrease as patient length of stay increases.[6]

# Pricing for Selected Outpatient Services

Medicare implemented a prospective payment system (PPS) for outpatient services in August 2000.[1] Different service bundles are classified under about 800 ambulatory payment classification groups (APCs). Each APC contains clinically similar services with comparable resource use, and each is assigned a relative weight based on the median cost of the services included in the group. Roughly 350 APCs are for pharmaceuticals or devices. Eighty are reserved for new technologies for which Medicare does not yet have the reliable cost information needed to fold them into a regular APC.[2] Distinct from the outpatient PPS, ambulatory surgical centers now provide many services—including cataract surgery, colonoscopy, and arthroscopy—that once required hospitalization.[3]

A conversion factor transforms the APC weights into dollar payments. The outpatient conversion factor was $63.694 in 2008. It is increased annually by the increase in the hospital market basket index unless Congress stipulates otherwise. To account for geographic differences in input prices, Medicare adjusts the labor portion of the conversion factor (60 percent) by the hospital wage index. For extremely expensive cases, outlier payments cover half of costs that exceed 1.75 times the standard payment rate and that also exceed the payment rate by $1,575. As with inpatient services, some hospitals have abused this provision.[4] Certain items involving new technologies—drugs, biologicals, and implantable devices—are not encompassed by the technology-related APCs and are paid separately.[5]

Clinical laboratory fees are handled differently. In theory, Medicare pays prospectively set fees for clinical lab services. In practice, however, 98 percent of lab tests are paid on the basis of national limits. Each Medicare payment region has a separate fee schedule. Each fee schedule covers over 1,100 separate tests or combinations of tests. Prices are based on 1983 laboratory charges adjusted for subsequent inflation. The national payment limits are set at 74 percent of the median amounts in the various regional fee schedules.

Medicare pays rental fees or purchase costs for durable medical equipment according to fee schedules for over 2,000 product groups. Payments are increased annually by the change in the consumer price index. Because Medicare payments for some equipment came to exceed prices paid by other buyers, in 1997 Congress authorized Medicare to freeze or cut payments and to conduct demonstrations to test the feasibility and implications for access and quality of setting payment rates through competitive bidding. The demonstrations found that competitive bidding reduced costs by about 20 percent with no serious quality or access issues.[6] As a result, the Medicare Modernization Act (MMA) instructed Medicare to phase in a competitive bidding system for most durable medical equipment products in large urban markets between 2008 and 2009.[7]

Dialysis fees are slightly higher for hospital-based facilities than for the 4,200 free-standing centers, but are the same for hemodialysis and peritoneal dialysis. A base prospective payment is adjusted crudely for differences in case mix and local input prices.[8] Facilities also receive separate payments for certain new injectable drugs and vitamins and lab tests, possibly creating a strong incentive to provide these separately billed drugs.[9] They now account for about 35 percent of the payments made to facilities.

Several dialysis quality measures, including the share of patients who received adequate dialysis and whose anemia was under control, improved from 2000 to 2005.[10] Because the number of surviving patients is growing, dialysis-related payments have increased rapidly and accounted for about 2 percent of Medicare's expenditures in 2006.

## Appendix C
# Sustainable Growth Rate System

The sustainable growth rate (SGR) system links the growth of per beneficiary spending on physician services to a complex index based on the prices that physicians are paid and changes in the following factors: Medicare fee-for-service enrollment, per capita gross domestic product, law or regulation, and estimated physician productivity. Because the physician payment update is tied to economic growth, the relationship between the growth in costs and payments is weak. And because the SGR formula adjusts for past estimating errors in economic growth and Medicare physician expenditures, the difference between the growth in costs and payments can be large.[1]

How this index translates into price per unit of service depends on the change in the quantity and character of medical services. If the quantity and intensity of services grow at the same rate as the statutorily permitted increase in total payments, then the conversion factor increases by the estimated change in the Medicare economic index (MEI), which is the measure of input price inflation for physician services publicly released by Medicare. Specifically, the MEI measures changes in the cost of physicians' time and operating expenses; it is a weighted sum of the prices of inputs in those two categories. Most of the components of the index come from the Bureau of Labor Statistics. Changes in the cost of physicians' time are measured using changes in nonfarm labor costs. Changes in "all-factor" productivity are also incorporated into the index as a way of accounting for improvements in physicians' productivity. The productivity adjustment to the MEI reduces its rate of growth.

If the quantity and intensity of services grows faster than the statutorily permitted increase in total payments, then the conversion factor is cut. Very rapid growth of quantity and intensity triggers correspondingly large price cuts. To forestall excessive reductions, Congress limited them to 5 percent. Without this provision, the SGR mechanism would have called for conversion factor price cuts of 26.7 percent in 2008. Any additions prevented by this limit are carried forward to be applied in later years.

Fees were actually cut by 4.8 percent in 2002. The formula called for a 4.4 percent cut in 2003 and still larger reductions in 2004 through 2009, but Congress responded to pressure from physicians and raised fees slightly or froze them each year over this period. Like Saint Augustine, Congress pledged fiscal virtue, but not just yet. The Deficit Reduction Act froze the 2006 conversion factor, but refinements to the relative value units resulted in an update of 0.2 percent. For 2007, the Tax Relief and Health Care Act effectively held payments at 2006 levels through a conversion factor bonus. The act provided a one-year 5 percent bonus to offset the 5 percent cut in the 2007 conversion factor as directed by the SGR and required that the 2008 conversion factor be calculated as if the bonus had never applied. The Medicare, Medicaid, and SCHIP Extension Act of 2007 postponed the scheduled reduction of fees of 10.1 percent for 2008 by six months and similarly specified that the conversion factor for the remainder of 2008 and subsequent years be computed as if the legislated increase for the first half of 2008 had never applied.

# Hospital Service Prices

As explained in chapter 2, Medicare's prospective payments for inpatient and outpatient hospital services are tied to a complex system of diagnosis-based categories. Controversy surrounds the number and definition of these categories.

## Complexity

Not only are Medicare payments linked to a large number of diagnosis-related groups (DRGs), but each DRG is composed of assorted conditions drawn from the International Classification of Diseases (Clinical Modification), which lists more than 11,500 distinct diseases and conditions.[1] Each condition may be manifested in patients whose co-morbidities, age, genetic inheritance, personal tastes for medical care, and physical state indicate treatment that differs in amount and in kind from that on which the payment category is based. As a result, actual costs within each payment category vary widely at any given point in time. Furthermore, they change at different rates over time as a result of learning-by-doing and small changes in technology that raise or lower treatment costs, but that Medicare may not recognize by amending DRG payments. Not every provider has the same mix of cases and patients. Consequently, some providers are paid too much and others too little, although outlier payments help match payments to actual incurred costs.

Modest increases in the number of payment categories would ameliorate this problem, but not much. In 2000 the Medicare Payment Advisory Commission found that increasing the number of DRGs from 500 to 900 would reduce the standard deviation of the gap between payments and incurred costs by only 5–10 percent and would further complicate administration.[2] It would also harm at least one key constituency—small and rural hospitals, which typically handle lower-cost cases within each DRG. These facilities constantly struggle for financial viability because they have few occupied beds over which to spread overhead costs. Linking DRG payments more accurately to costs would cut payments to rural hospitals and complicate their struggle for financial survival. Nonetheless, in 2008 Medicare began a two-year transition to a new system of 744 severity-adjusted diagnosis-related groups (Medicare Severity DRGs, or MS-DRGs) to replace the previous system of 538 DRGs.[3] Rural hospitals are expected to experience payment cuts between 0.5 and 1.8 percent in 2008, whereas urban, teaching, and disproportionate share hospitals (DSH) stand to gain 0.9 percent on average.[4]

## Controversy

Not surprisingly, some providers are discontented with prospective payment rates. The average costs of efficient providers are extraordinarily difficult to measure. Fixed and shared costs, such as management's salaries or equipment used for many services, vary from one provider to another. So does the number of services among which they must somehow be allocated. Such allocations are inescapably arbitrary. The average cost of providing a service efficiently varies depending on the size and location of the provider, the volume of services supplied by the facility, and the characteristics of patients served. Not all hospitals are equally efficient. Medicare tries to consider such factors, including labor costs, when it sets payments for individual facilities. But not all factors can be taken into account, and for some this imperfection can impose significant financial strain.

## DRG-Induced Distortions

The prospective payment system (PPS) fixed one problem. It ended the incentive—endemic in the cost-based reimbursement system it replaced—

to pad revenues by providing care of marginal worth. But prospective payment created other problems.

First, providers can improve their margins by stinting on care or by shunning cases expected to cost more than the anticipated fee. Medicare administrators tried to address this issue by providing "outlier" payments for exceptionally costly cases. But to determine the cost thresholds that define "outliers" and the amount above these thresholds Medicare will pay, administrators must make technically difficult and controversial tradeoffs.[5]

Second, Medicare also overpays for some DRGs. Some payments were set too high to start with, and some have fallen. However overpayments came to exist, entrepreneurial physicians and other investors have an incentive to set up hospitals that specialize in providing just these overpriced services, orthopedic surgery being one. Such hospitals may be quite profitable precisely because Medicare pays too much for some services and too little for others. The profits that specialty hospitals earn come at the expense of multiservice hospitals that would otherwise use profits from overpriced DRGs to cover losses on underpriced DRGs and to pay for uncompensated care. Thus specialty hospitals erode the capacity of multiservice hospitals to care for the uninsured or to serve patients with conditions for which reimbursements do not cover costs. Their owners point to solid evidence that quality of care tends to be highest in facilities that perform certain surgeries at least a minimum number of times each year. Indeed, one Medicare strategy to raise the quality of care is to encourage the concentration of certain procedures in so-called Centers of Excellence. Given the rapid change in medical technology, the learning curve associated with new medical procedures, and the difficulty of setting prices correctly, this problem is likely to remain serious as long as specialty hospitals are permitted. Congress recognized this problem in 2003 when it imposed an eighteen-month moratorium that effectively halted the development of new physician-owned specialty hospitals.[6] Legislation considered in 2007 would permanently limit physician ownership in and referral to these facilities.[7]

## Unbundling

Paying a flat sum for a "bundle" of services may also encourage hospitals, nursing homes, home health agencies, dialysis centers, and physicians to "unbundle" services in a way that secures two payments rather than one. For example, the DRG payment that covers hospital costs of treating stroke victims includes the anticipated cost of speech therapy. But if the patient is transferred to a skilled nursing facility (SNF) or sent home, the hospital saves the costs of speech therapy and other recuperative services, and the SNF or home health agency receives an additional payment for providing them. Such transfers sometimes achieve genuine savings. Patients requiring only speech therapy do not need all of the costly backup services available at a full-service hospital. Transferring such patients sacrifices no medical benefit and saves money. These transfers should be encouraged by allowing providers to retain part of the savings. But cost reductions from providing care in separate and less costly settings should not trigger increases in total payments.

To deal with this problem, Medicare in 1999 began to cut DRG payments for ten conditions if patients received care from a posacute care facility that could have been part of their inpatient treatment regimen. Providers objected strongly to this reform and have lobbied Congress to deny the secretary of the Department of Health and Human Services authority to expand the initiative. Nonetheless, Medicare subsequently expanded payment cuts for all patients transferred to another hospital covered under the inpatient PPS, for patients transferred to postacute care settings with one of 182 particular DRGs, and for those with a hospital length of stay at least one day less than the average stay for their DRG.[8]

Setting one price for bundles of services creates an additional problem for both providers and Medicare when technology advances rapidly. Providers would like to bill separately for new and expensive devices, drugs, and procedures. They correctly argue that Medicare's payments do not cover the high costs of many innovations. If providers use the innovation, they lose money. If they do not, patients may receive suboptimal care. Medicare has tried to deal with this dilemma for outpatient services by defining ambulatory payment classes for new technologies and by allowing pass-through payments for drugs, biologicals, and devices that are inadequately reflected in the payment rates.[9] Similarly, dialysis centers are permitted to bill separately for injectable drugs and laboratory tests that in recent years have become increasingly important components of modern treatment. Understandably, providers fight to expand and extend the scope of these special payments even when the underlying costs have been reflected in the payment rates.

As noted in the text, the difficulties in setting hospital prices are not unique to Medicare: all other insurers face the same challenges. In fact, it is a common practice for private insurers to use Medicare payment systems wholly or as a point of reference in setting their own prices.

# Notes

## Chapter 1

1. The effects were largest for nonemergency procedures. This category now includes joint replacements and coronary artery bypass surgery. Average effects on health status are modest, but largest for those groups that experienced the greatest increases in insurance coverage. See David E. Card, Carlos Dobkin, and Nicole Maestas, "The Impact of Nearly Universal Insurance Coverage on Health Care Utilization and Health: Evidence from Medicare," Working Paper W10365 (Cambridge, Mass.: National Bureau of Economic Research, March 2004). These results are similar to those found with respect to universal coverage in Canada. See Sandra L. Decker and Dahlia Remler, "How Much Might Universal Health Insurance Reduce Socioeconomic Disparities in Health? A Comparison of the U.S. and Canada," Working Paper W10715 (Cambridge, Mass.: National Bureau of Economic Research, August 2004).

2. David Card, Carlos Dobkin, and Nicole Maestas, "Does Medicare Save Lives?" Working Paper 13668 (Cambridge, Mass.: National Bureau of Economic Research, November 2007) (www.nber.org/papers/w13668).

3. Institute of Medicine, *To Err Is Human: Building a Safer Health Care System* (Washington: National Academy of Science, 1999); Elizabeth McGlynn and others, "The Quality of Health Care Delivered to Adults in the United States," *New England Journal of Medicine* 348 (June 2003): 2635–45.

4. "Johnson Signs Medicare," *Kansas City Times,* July 31, 1965; Doris Kearns Goodwin, *Lyndon Johnson and the American Dream* (New York: Harper and Row, 1976), p. 250.

5. John D. Morris, "President Signs Medicare Bill: Praises Truman," *New York Times,* July 31, 1965, pp. 1, 8.

6. Eric Goldman, *The Tragedy of Lyndon Johnson* (New York: Knopf, 1969), p. 291; and *Congressional Record*, February 9, 1965, p. 2421.

7. Goldman, *The Tragedy of Lyndon Johnson*, pp. 288–89.

8. Robert Dallek, *Lyndon B. Johnson: Portrait of a President* (Oxford University Press, 2004), p. 199.

9. David A. Hyman, *Medicare Meets Mephistopheles* (Washington: Cato Institute, 2006).

10. H.R. 6675, "The Mills Bill," formally enacted as the Social Security Amendments of 1965 (P.L. 88-97). Final House vote, July 27, 1965: voting yes, 237 Democrats, 70 Republicans; voting no, 47 Democrats, 69 Republicans; not voting, 8 Democrats, 2 Republicans. Final Senate vote, July 28, 1965: voting yes, 57 Democrats, 13 Republicans; voting no, 7 Democrats, 17 Republicans; not voting, 4 Democrats, 2 Republicans.

11. Robert J. Myers, *Actuarial Cost Estimates and Summary of Provisions of the Old Age, Survivors, and Disability Insurance System as Modified by the Social Security Amendments of 1965, and Actuarial Cost Estimates and Summary of Provisions of the Hospital Insurance and Supplementary Medical Insurance Systems Established by Such Act*, prepared for House Committee on Ways and Means, 89 Cong. 1 sess. (U.S. Government Printing Office, July 30, 1965). Figure increased from 1967 to 2007 dollars using historical, annual consumer price index changes from 1967 to 2007. The index measures changes in prices of all goods and services purchased for consumption by urban households.

12. On the history of this legislation, see Sandra Christensen and Rick Kasten, "Covering Catastrophic Expenses under Medicare," *Health Affairs* 7 (Winter 1988): 79–93; Thomas Rice, Katherine Desmond, and Jon Gabel, "The Medicare Catastrophic Coverage Act: A Post Mortem," *Health Affairs* 9 (Fall 1990): 75–87; and Jonathan Oberlander, *The Political Life of Medicare* (University of Chicago Press, 2003).

13. On the history of this period, see Elizabeth Drew, *Showdown: The Struggle between the Gingrich Congress and Clinton White House* (New York: Simon and Schuster, 1996); David G. Smith, *Entitlement Politics: Medicare and Medicaid, 1995–2001* (Edison, N.J.: Transaction, 2002).

14. Federal Hospital Insurance (FHI) Board of Trustees, *1997 Annual Report of the Board of Trustees of the Federal Hospital Insurance Trust Fund* (1997).

15. The major pieces of legislation were the Balanced Budget Refinement Act of 1999 (BBRA, P.L. 106-113), and the Medicare, Medicaid and SCHIP Benefits Improvement and Protection Act of 2000 (BIPA, P.L. 106-554).

16. FHI Board of Trustees, *2001 Annual Report of the Board of Trustees of the Federal Hospital Insurance and Federal Supplementary Medical Insurance Trust Funds* (2001).

17. See Section 401 ("Reserve Fund for Medicare Modernization and Prescription Drugs") in H. Con. Res. 95, "Establishing the congressional budget for the United States Government for fiscal year 2004 and setting forth appropriate budgetary levels for fiscal years 2003 and 2005 through 2013," 108 Cong. 1 sess. (agreed to April 11, 2003) (http://frwebgate.access.gpo.gov/cgi-bin/getdoc.cgi?dbname=108_cong_bills&docid=f:hc95enr.txt.pdf).

18. At 5:50 a.m. on November 22, 2003, the House approved the conference report (H. Rept. 1) 220-215 (voting yes, 204 Republicans, 16 Democrats; voting no, 25 Republicans, 189 Democrats, and 1 Independent). This was the longest known roll-call vote in the history of the House. Members reported that they had never witnessed such intense pressure and arm twisting. For a review of its passage, see Thomas R. Oliver, Philip R. Lee, and

Helene L. Lipton, "A Political History of Medicare and Prescription Drug Coverage," *Milbank Quarterly* 82 (June 2004): 283–354; and John K. Iglehart, "The New Medicare Prescription-Drug Benefit: A Pure Power Play," *New England Journal of Medicine* 350 (February 2004): 826–33.

19. The Senate approved the conference report 54-44 (voting yes, 42 Republicans, 11 Democrats, and 1 Independent; voting no, 9 Republicans, 35 Democrats; not voting, 2 Democrats).

20. For a summary of the MMA, see Kaiser Family Foundation and Health Policy Alternatives, Inc., "Prescription Drug Coverage for Medicare Beneficiaries: An Overview of the Medicare Prescription Drug, Improvement, and Modernization Act of 2003 (Public Law 108-173)" (Menlo Park, Calif., 2004) (www.kff.org/medicare/upload/Prescription-Drug-Coverage-for-Medicare-Beneficiares-An-Overview-of-the-Medicare-Prescription-Drug-Improvement-Act-2003.pdf).

21. This charge triggered both an investigation by the House Select Committee on Standards of Official Conduct and a probe by the Federal Bureau of Investigation. American Health Line, March 26 and June 22, 2004; "GOP Leaders Threaten Smith's Son's Campaign over Medicare Vote," Associated Press, November 24, 2003 (www.campaignlegalcenter.org/attachments/964.pdf).

22. Rick Foster, Testimony before the Committee on Ways and Means, March 24, 2004. This charge triggered investigations by the Justice Department and the Inspector General of the Department of Health and Human Services (IG-HHS) and analyses by the Congressional Research Service (CRS) and the Government Accountability Office (GAO). The IG-HHS judgment was that the CMS administrator was within his rights to withhold the estimates from Congress, but CRS concluded that the action was "probably illegal," and the GAO ruled that because he violated an arcane provision of an appropriation act, the administrator's salary should have been withheld. Jack Maskell (CRS), letter to Charles Rangel, subject: "Agency Prohibiting a Federal Officer from Providing Accurate Cost Information to the United States Congress," April 26, 2004 (www.fas.org/sgp/crs/crs042604.pdf). Also Office of the Inspector General, Department of Health and Human Services, July 6, 2004 (http://oig.hhs.gov/publications/docs/press/2004/070704IGStatement.pdf); GAO Letter B-302911 to Senator Frank R. Lautenberg and others, "Department of Health and Human Services—Chief Actuary's Communications with Congress," September 7, 2004 (http://lautenberg.senate.gov/ images/B-302911.pdf).

23. It was charged, for example, that the announcements mentioned a $35 monthly premium when this amount was not guaranteed by the legislation and CMS estimated a $37.23 premium, that the message was being conveyed by an actor portraying herself as a news reporter, and that the president was receiving credit for what was a joint effort of Congress and the executive branch.

24. Karen Davis and others, "Medicare versus Private Insurance: Rhetoric and Reality" *Health Affairs*, Web Exclusive (October 9, 2002): W311-24.

25. Congressional Budget Office (CBO), *The Long-Term Outlook for Health Care Spending* (November 2007).

26. Calculated from supplemental data published with the CBO, *The Long-Term Budget Outlook* (December 2007) (www.cbo.gov/ftpdocs/88xx/doc8877/SupplementalData.xls). Medicare outlays are net of offsetting receipts.

27. The increase in the deficit resulting from the MMA is nearly two times the projected gap between Social Security spending and revenues. The Medicare and Social Security trustees estimate the seventy-five-year unfunded obligations of Part D and OASDI (present value of future cost less future taxes through 2082, reduced by the amount of trust fund assets at the beginning of 2008) at $7.9 trillion and $4.3 trillion, respectively. See FHI Board of Trustees, *2008 Annual Report of the Board of Trustees of the Federal Hospital Insurance and Federal Supplementary Medical Insurance Trust Funds* (2008), table III.C23 ("Unfunded Part D Obligations from Program Inception through the Infinite Horizon"); and FHI Board of Trustees, *2008 Annual Report of the Board of Trustees of the Federal Old-Age and Survivors Insurance and Federal Disability Insurance Trust Funds* (2008), table IV.B6 ("Unfunded OASDI Obligations for 1935 through the Infinite Horizon"). President Bush and others have labeled the Social Security shortfall a "train wreck." See White House, Office of the Press Secretary, "President Participates in Social Security Conversation in Indiana," March 4, 2005 (www.whitehouse.gov/news/releases/2005/03/20050304-15.html).

28. Liqun Liu, Andrew J. Rettenmaier, and Zijun Wang, "The Rising Burden of Health Spending on Seniors" (Washington: National Center for Policy Analysis, February 2007).

29. Kaiser Family Foundation, *Medicare Chart Book, 2005* (Menlo Park, Calif., 2005) (www.kff.org/medicare/upload/Medicare-Chart-Book-3rd-Edition-Summer-2005-Section-4.pdf).

30. Financial Accounting Standards Board, Summary of Statement 106, "Employers' Accounting for Postretirement Benefits Other than Pensions" (issued December 1990) (www.fasb.org/st/summary/stsum106.shtml).

31. Kaiser Family Foundation and the Health Research and Educational Trust, *Employer Health Benefits 2007* (Menlo Park, Calif., 2007) (www.kff.org/insurance/7672/sections/ehbs07-sec11-1.cfm).

32. Kaiser Family Foundation and Hewitt Associates, *Retiree Health Benefits Examined: Findings from the Kaiser/Hewitt 2006 Survey on Retiree Health Benefits* (Menlo Park, Calif., 2006) (www.kff.org/medicare/upload/7587.pdf).

# Chapter 2

1. Lawmakers modeled the Part A benefit on the standard Blue Cross hospitalization plan and the Part B benefit on the medical services plan offered to federal workers by Aetna Insurance Company.

2. To be eligible, those with end-stage renal disease must be workers who participate in the Social Security system or must be the spouse or dependent of an eligible worker.

3. Federal Hospital Insurance (FHI) Board of Trustees, *2008 Annual Report of the Board of Trustees of the Federal Hospital Insurance and Federal Supplementary Medical Insurance Trust Funds* (2008), tables III.A3 and IV.B5. About half of those with renal failure are disabled. Those sixty-five and older with kidney failure are included with the elderly. The number of disabled beneficiaries has quadrupled since 1973, but only 47 percent of Americans aged sixteen to sixty-four with a severe disability are covered by Medicare. Author's calculations, based on U.S. Bureau of the Census, *Disability Selected Characteristics of Persons 16 to 74: 2005* (2005), table 1 (www.census.gov/hhes/www/disability/cps/cps105.html).

4. Does not include premiums as offsetting receipts. FHI Board of Trustees, *2008 Annual Report*, table II.B1.

5. U.S. Bureau of the Census, *Statistical Abstract of the United States 1967* (1967), p. 73, reports that of those sixty-five and older in 1962–63, 54.0 percent had some hospital insurance and 45.7 percent had some surgical insurance.

6. Ninety-nine percent of those sixty-five and older have Part A coverage. Those without ten years of covered employment may buy coverage at an actuarially fair premium, costing $5,076 a year in 2008. The premium is reduced to $2,796 a year for people with seven and one-half to ten years of covered employment.

7. Certain low-income beneficiaries are automatically enrolled in Part D if they do not join a plan on their own. Otherwise, enrollment in Medicare drug plans is voluntary. However, unless beneficiaries have drug coverage at least as good as the standard Medicare drug benefit (known as "creditable coverage"), those who join a plan after their initial eligibility enrollment period will pay a penalty equal to 1 percent of the national base beneficiary premium ($27.93 in 2008) for each month they delayed enrollment, for as long as they are enrolled in a Medicare drug plan.

8. By law, Part B premiums are set at 25 percent of the expected program cost for those sixty-five and older. Some 3 million people are enrolled in Part A but not Part B and are mainly elderly or disabled individuals who are still working and have primary health insurance coverage through an employer-sponsored health insurance plan. They decline Part B coverage because it does not offer additional protections above what they obtain from their work-related plan. They may enroll in Part B when they lose their work-related insurance. In addition, approximately 400,000 people receive Part B but not Part A benefits. For the most part, this group consists of older retirees who worked for the federal government and state and local governments and did not contribute to Social Security. Although not entitled to Part A, they may still join Part B.

9. Along with the carrots, a stick encourages Part B participation: those who do not enroll in Part B when first eligible and who do not have employer-sponsored coverage face increased monthly premiums should they decide to join the program later. The lifetime penalty is a 10 percent higher premium for every twelve months by which enrollment is delayed.

10. For fiscal 2008, the income threshold was updated to $82,000 for individuals and $164,000 for couples. When fully implemented in 2011, Part B premiums paid by high-income Medicare enrollees—defined in 2008 as single persons with incomes over $205,000 and couples with incomes over $410,000—will cover 80 percent of the program's average costs per beneficiary.

11. Centers for Medicare and Medicaid Services (CMS), *Fact Sheet: Medicare Premiums and Deductibles for 2007* (September 12, 2006).

12. Medicare offers the widest provider network possible. Moreover, it pays for services at lower rates on average than those paid by private insurers; has low administrative and marketing costs, no costs for insurance reserves, and no need for profits; guarantees issue; and charges all participants premiums based on average costs.

13. Medicare Advantage has been renamed several times. The option was first offered in 1982 by the Tax Equity and Fiscal Responsibility Act, and the plans were known as TEFRA HMOs or Medicare HMOs. The Balanced Budget Act of 1997 renamed the option Medicare+Choice (M+C). In 2003 the Medicare Modernization Act changed the name to

Medicare Advantage. The range of allowed plans has grown, and the method of determining the capitated payments to the plans has been revised. For simplicity, we refer to this option as Medicare Advantage throughout these periods.

14. MA enrollees must continue to pay Medicare Part B premiums. They may disenroll from MA or change plans once during a six-month period. Before 2006, beneficiaries could enroll or disenroll at any time. Michigan Poverty Law Program Newsletter, "New Medicare Fee Schedule and Medicare Eligibility Rules for 2007," no. 32, Winter 2007; Kaiser Family Foundation, "Medicare Advantage Fact Sheet" (Menlo Park, Calif., September 2005).

15. Kaiser Family Foundation, Medicare Chart Book, 2005 (Menlo Park, Calif., 2005) (www.kff.org/medicare/upload/Medicare-Chart-Book-3rd-Edition-Summer-2005-Section-4.pdf).

16. Together, all inpatient hospital services accounted for 29 percent of Medicare spending in 2006, down from 45 percent in 1996. Medicare represents about 40 percent of inpatient hospital revenue. Medicare Payment Advisory Commission (MedPAC), *A Data Book: Healthcare Spending and the Medicare Program* (June 2007), p. 9; MedPAC, *Report to the Congress: Medicare Payment Policy* (March 2008), p. 54.

17. Medicare provides similar coverage in hospitals that specialize in the treatment of cancer, children's illnesses, psychiatric conditions, and long-term care, and in hospital-like facilities, such as inpatient rehabilitation facilities.

18. There are actually 746 categories; 2 are not used for payment. In 2008 Medicare began a two-year transition to a system of severity-adjusted DRGs known as Medicare severity (MS) DRGs. The new system has 335 base DRGs that reflect similar principal diagnoses and procedures. Most base DRGs are further subdivided on the basis of whether patients have no complication or co-morbidity (CC), one or more CCs, or one or more major CCs. In the first year, payments will be based on a 50/50 blend of MS-DRGs and the previous DRGs. MedPAC, *Medicare Payment Basics: Hospital Acute Inpatient Services Payment System* (October 2007). The DRG concept has been extended beyond inpatient hospital care: in 2008 there were 796 payment categories for ambulatory care, 153 for home health care, and 53 for nursing home care. DRG payments vary enormously. The DRG price for the most costly procedure, heart transplant or implant of heart assist system with a major co-morbidity or complication, is 150 times that of the least costly, medication for a normal newborn. The most common DRG in 2004 was heart failure and shock, which accounted for 6 percent of discharges in that year. The ten most common DRGs in 2004 accounted for 30 percent of all discharges and 21 percent of payments at hospitals paid under the prospective payment system. CMS, "FY 2008 Final Rule: List of MS-DRGs, Relative Weighting Factors, and Geometric and Arithmetic Mean Length of Stay," Acute Inpatient Prospective Payment System (PPS), Acute Inpatient Files (Baltimore: December 2007) (www.cms.hhs.gov/AcuteInpatientPPS/downloads/WI_TABLES_FY_2008_Final_Rule.zip); and MedPAC, *A Data Book: Healthcare Spending and the Medicare Program* (June 2006), p. 78.

19. Discharges are categorized into DRGs on the basis of patients' sex, age, clinical conditions, and treatment strategies. Clinical conditions are defined by patients' primary discharge diagnosis and up to eight supplementary diagnoses. The treatment strategy—surgical or medical—can vary from one to six procedures during the stay. The exact payment is based on two factors: a standardized or base payment amount and a weight that measures the costliness of each DRG in relation to the average DRG. The base payment

amount, which is updated annually, has separate operating and capital cost components. In 2008 the standardized operating payment was $4,964 and the capital component $423. MedPAC, *Medicare Payment Basics: Hospital Acute Inpatient Services.* The area with highest labor costs in 2008, Santa Cruz, California, was more than twice as expensive as the area with lowest costs, rural North Dakota. Wages in Santa Cruz were 62 (*78*) percent higher than the national urban (*rural*) average; those in rural North Dakota were 24 (*18*) percent lower than the national urban (*rural*) average. The geographic wage index is applied to the labor-related portion of the base rate, which reflects an estimate of the portion of costs affected by local wage rates and fringe benefits. Medicare's current estimate of the operating labor share is 69.7 percent. The MMA lowered this fraction to 62 percent for areas with a wage index less than or equal to 1.0 in an effort to boost payments to nonmetropolitan hospitals. CMS, "FY 2008 Final Rule."

20. Outlier payments are intended to reduce any incentive hospitals may have to shun cases that are likely to be very costly. Outlier payments offset 80 percent of the extraordinary costs for patients whose care costs far more than the payment rate for their DRGs. Costs that exceed the sum of the DRG payment (both operating and capital), a fixed loss amount ($22,635 for 2008), and any indirect medical education, disproportionate share, or new technology payments qualify for outlier payments. In 2005 these payments applied to only 2 percent of discharges but accounted for 4 percent of total payments. In recent years, some hospitals have illegally abused the complex outlier rules in an effort to gain extra revenues. MedPAC, *Report to the Congress: Medicare Payment Policy* (March 2007).

21. Payments for direct costs of medical education vary with the number of residents, the historic cost per resident, and the proportion of a hospital's patient days represented by Medicare patients. Per resident payments are frozen for hospitals with amounts above 140 percent of the national average. Payments for indirect costs of medical education vary with the number of a hospital's residents per bed. They are intended to cover the extra tests and procedures residents commonly prescribe. For 2008, the operating indirect medical education adjustment will increase to 5.5 for every 10 percent increase in the resident-to-bed ratio and then stay at this level in subsequent years. MedPAC, *Medicare Payment Basics: Hospital Acute Inpatient Services.*

22. These so-called disproportionate share payments are based on the excess over 15 percent of a hospital's share of low-income patients. A hospital's low-income share is the sum of the proportion of its Medicare inpatient days provided to persons eligible for Supplemental Security Income benefits and the proportion of its total acute inpatient days furnished to Medicaid patients. These payments vary by hospital size, urban/rural location, and whether the hospital is the only one in a geographic area. The relationship between such payments and uncompensated care is tenuous.

23. About 20 percent of PPS hospitals are covered by three special payment provisions intended to help rural facilities that do not become critical-access hospitals: rural referral (RRCs), sole community (SCHs), and small rural Medicare-dependent hospitals (MDHs). These facilities provide about 11 percent of all discharges under the PPS. MedPAC, *A Data Book* (2007), p. 73. The RRC program was established to support high-volume rural hospitals that treat a large number of complicated cases. Rural hospitals that have at least 275 beds or meet other criteria, including having a case-mix index and discharge rate equal to or greater than the median number for urban hospitals in that census region, can be classified as RRCs. To qualify for the SCH program, a hospital must be located at least 35 miles

from the nearest like hospital (excluding critical-access hospitals) or meet other federal criteria for being deemed a community's sole source of care. To qualify for MDH designation, a facility must be located in a rural area, have no more than 100 beds, not be classified as an SCH, and have at least 60 percent of inpatient days or admissions attributable to Medicare patients. RRCs are paid on the basis of the urban, rather than rural, prospective payment rates as adjusted by the applicable DRG weighting factor and the rural area index. SCHs receive the higher of either (a) standard inpatient prospective payment rates or (b) payments based on the hospital's costs in a base year updated to the current year and adjusted for changes in their case mix. MDHs are similar, but they are eligible for a prospective payment rate blend of current PPS rates (25 percent) and their historical costs (75 percent). MedPAC, *Medicare Payment Basics: Critical Access Hospitals Payment System* (October 2007).

24. Before 2006, small hospitals with twenty-five or fewer beds could convert to critical access (CAH) status if they were (a) 35 miles by primary road, (b) 15 miles by secondary road from the nearest hospital, or (c) their state waived the distance requirement by declaring the hospital a "necessary provider." After 2006 states could no longer waive the distance requirement. While about 65 percent of existing CAHs fail the distance test, they are grandfathered into the program. Among small rural hospitals that have not converted, most would not meet the distance requirement. Unlike SCHs and MDHs, which only receive cost-based payments for inpatient care, CAHs operate outside of the PPS and receive cost-based payments for inpatient, outpatient, lab, therapy, and postacute services in swing beds. CAHs represent 24 percent of all short-stay hospitals but account for only 3 percent of all discharges. MedPAC, *Medicare Payment Basics: Critical Access Hospitals;* and MedPAC, *A Data Book* (2007), p. 73.

25. In 2006, 5.5 percent of Medicare spending went for outpatient services in hospitals and surgical centers, with 6 percent going to services delivered by about 3,500 facilities in the hospital outpatient PPS, and 0.5 percent to services provided by 4,707 ambulatory surgical centers (ASCs). Medicare outpatient payments that year accounted for 15 percent of hospital payments. FHI Board of Trustees, *2008 Annual Report*, table II.B1; MedPAC, *A Data Book* (2007), pp. 110, 116. Medicare's proportion of payment for these services increased from 60 percent in 2001, the first full year of the outpatient PPS, to about 70 percent in 2006. For many years, Medicare allowed hospitals to charge patients 20 percent of the "reasonable and customary" fee for the services they received. Although that 20 percent was based on a patient's total allowable income, Medicare used a complex formula that generated a much lower number from which to determine its 80 percent of the fees. As a result, patients were actually responsible for close to half of the cost on average. For some services, such as electrocardiograms, the patient paid more than 75 percent of the cost. In 1997, 1999, and 2000, Congress adopted reforms to control the growth of charges for outpatient services and to gradually bring patient financial exposure down to 20 percent of total payments. In the prospective payment system implemented in 2000, the nominal amounts for outpatient care could be frozen if they exceeded 20 percent of the amounts set in the fee schedule. As annual adjustments push up the prospective payment amounts, the share of total payments borne by patients will fall, but CMS has estimated that it could take three to four decades before the coinsurance for all procedures reaches 20 percent. MedPAC, *Report to the Congress: Medicare Payment Policy* (March 2001), pp. 142, 145; MedPAC, *A Data Book* (2007), p. 109.

26. In 2008 Medicare began a four-year transition to a new payment system for ASCs based on the hospital outpatient PPS. The ASC conversion factor will be based on a percentage of the OPPS conversion factor.

27. Medicare pays for four categories of hospice care: routine home care, continuous home care, inpatient respite care, and general inpatient care. Routine home care accounts for about 95 percent of all care. Inpatient care cannot exceed one-fifth of the care delivered by an agency. Payments are adjusted for geographic differences in labor costs and are updated annually by the same percent as inpatient hospital payments. The aggregate payment to each hospice is subject to an annual limit that varies with the number of beneficiaries newly enrolled during the year. The labor-related fractions of the payments that are adjusted are 69 percent for routine and continuous home care, 54 percent for inpatient respite care, and 64 percent for general inpatient care. The cap on payments for 2007 was $21,410 multiplied by the number of beneficiaries newly enrolled during the year.

28. MedPAC, *Report to the Congress: Increasing the Value of Medicare* (June 2006), p. 65. The total cost in 2007 was $10 billion, about 2.5 percent of Medicare spending in that year. James Matthews, "Hospice Costs and Payments," prepared for MedPAC (March 2008) (www.medpac.gov/transcripts/20080306_hospice_FNL.pdf).

29. Diane Campbell and others, "Medicare Program Expenditures Associated with Hospice Use," *Annals of Internal Medicine* 140 (February 2004): 269–77.

30. The most common diagnosis for an SNF admission in 2005 was a major joint and limb reattachment procedure of the lower extremity (typically a hip or knee replacement). The ten most frequent conditions accounted for about 37 percent of all SNF admissions. Freestanding, hospital-based, for-profit, and nonprofit facilities had the same top ten diagnoses, although the rank orderings of the top four conditions differed slightly. MedPAC, *Report to the Congress: Medicare Payment Policy* (2008), p. 145.

31. After 20 days, beneficiaries pay a co-payment set at one-eighth of the hospital deductible—$128 a day in 2008—which covers approximately two-fifths of the average daily cost of SNF care. The maximum liability a beneficiary faced in 2008 was $10,240 for the first 100 days of SNF care. In 1999 the Medicare SNF co-payment was $96, the average daily charge for all SNF residents was $115.91, and the charge for Medicare beneficiaries was $166.37. MedPAC, *Medicare Payment Basics: Skilled Nursing Facility Services Payment System* (October 2007); National Nursing Home Survey (1999), unpublished data.

32. The SNF co-payment does not vary geographically or by facility, although the cost of care varies widely. Even if the daily rate charged by an SNF is below the co-payment rate, the beneficiary must pay the co-payment. In fiscal 2007, 5 percent of Medicare's expenditures were for care delivered by some 15,000 SNFs. Medicare payments for skilled nursing care made up only 1 percent of the overall payments to hospitals in 2006. MedPAC, *Report to the Congress: Medicare Payment Policy* (2008), pp. 49, 145.

33. Patients are assigned to one of the fifty-three RUGs on the basis of patient characteristics and service use that are expected to require similar resources. The daily rate paid for each RUG is made up of a fixed amount for room, board, and other routine services and group-specific amounts reflecting the anticipated intensity of nursing needs and therapy use for each group. There are separate rates for urban and rural facilities, and payments are adjusted for local cost differences. The hospital wage index is used to adjust the 70 percent of costs that are estimated to be attributable to labor costs. SNF operators complained that the new fee system was too stringent. They also alleged that the new system could cause

access problems for patients suffering from Alzheimer's disease and other hard-to-care-for conditions. Congress responded by raising all payments temporarily and those for hard-to-serve patients permanently. MedPAC, *Medicare Payment Basics: Skilled Nursing Facility Services.*

34. About 2.9 million beneficiaries (or 8.1 percent of FFS beneficiaries) used home health care in 2006. Medicare home health payments constitute the preponderance of revenues of the nation's 9,200 home health agencies but accounted for only 3.2 percent of total Medicare spending in 2006. MedPAC, *Report to the Congress: Medicare Payment Policy* (2008), p. 174.

35. Homebound patients may receive skilled nursing, physical therapy, occupational therapy, speech therapy, aide service, and medical social work provided in their home on an intermittent basis. This group includes people who can only leave home with considerable effort and only with the aid of special devices such as a wheelchair.

36. Writing rules to distinguish people who "need" home health care services from those who do not has proved challenging. Such rules are bound to be somewhat arbitrary. Physicians and other providers in the field exercise considerable discretion, and their incentives often differ somewhat from those of policymakers and program administrators. Under current rules, eligible patients must need only "intermittent" care, which is defined as less than seven days of care a week or less than eight hours a day for less than twenty-one days. In one of the more important changes made by the Balanced Budget Act of 1997, eligibility for home health payments was denied if the only required service was for a skilled nurse to draw blood.

37. MedPAC, *Report to the Congress: Medicare Payment Policy* (March 2003), pp. 105–06.

38. Under the prospective payment system, patients are assigned to one of 153 home health resource groups (HHRGs) according to measures of patients' clinical and functional severity and the use of therapy during the home health episode. Home health agencies are paid fixed amounts for each sixty-day episode of home health care involving five or more visits. Payments for the various HHRGs are adjusted for differences in labor cost across areas. When the costs for providing services exceed the payment for an episode by more than 65 percent, outlier payments offset 80 percent of the costs above the threshold. The labor portion of the payment, 77 percent of the total, is adjusted by the hospital wage index. The average payment per episode was $2,569 in 2006. MedPAC, *Medicare Payment Basics: Home Health Care Services Payment System* (October 2007). MedPAC, *Report to the Congress: Medicare Payment Policy* (2008), p. 174.

39. Despite the restrictions on payments, the overall quality of home care has improved. An increased proportion of patients report less pain and are able to accomplish activities of daily living such as bathing or walking. The rate of use of the hospital or the emergency room during a home health episode has remained constant in conjunction with this improvement. MedPAC, *Report to the Congress: Medicare Payment Policy* (2008), p. 179.

40. Ibid., p. 174.

41. In rural areas, the proportion is even higher—40 percent. Center for Studying Health System Change, "Physician Incomes in Rural and Urban America" Issue Brief 92 (January 2005).

42. MedPAC, *A Data Book* (2007), p. 53.

43. CMS Fact Sheet, October 1, 2007. The deductible does not apply to home health services, prevention services, laboratory charges, flu shots, and community health center services. Coinsurance is not required for laboratory charges. The deductible increases each year at the same rate as Part B expenditures per aged beneficiary. The Medicare Modernization Act of 2003 (P.L. 108-173), sec. 629, made this change.

44. Separate fee schedules that are set at a fraction of the schedule for physicians govern payments to physician assistants and nurse practitioners, anesthetists and nurse anesthetists, psychologists, social workers, and physical therapists. Beneficiaries are responsible for 20 percent of their bills as well.

45. The proportion of physicians who "participate" varies by specialty and region, but in 2006, 93.3 percent of practicing physicians and more than 96.7 percent of allowed charges were associated with physicians who accepted Medicare's fees as payment in full. Only 0.6 percent of allowed charges were for services provided by nonparticipating physicians who also did not accept assignment. MedPAC, *Report to the Congress: Medicare Payment Policy* (2008), p. 88–89.

46. Nonparticipating physicians may choose on a patient-by-patient basis whether to charge more than the Medicare fee schedule allows. Medicare includes the names of participating physicians in directories it distributes to beneficiaries.

47. Specifically, Medicare paid the smallest of (1) the physician's actual charge for the service, (2) the customary charge defined as the median fee the physician charged for the service during the previous period, and (3) the prevailing charge, which was the 75th percentile of the median charges of all physicians in the locality for the service.

48. FHI Board of Trustees, *2007 Annual Report*, p. 96.

49. CMS initially utilized 74 measures for the 2007 Physician Quality Reporting Initiative (PQRI). The 2008 measure set includes 117 clinical quality measures and 2 structural measures, namely, the use of electronic health records and electronic prescribing technology. CMS, "Physician Quality Reporting Initiative" (www.cms.hhs.gov/PQRI).

50. The bonus is 1.5 percent, subject to a cap. All Medicare-enrolled eligible professionals may participate, regardless of whether they have signed a Medicare participation agreement to accept assignment on all claims.

51. The payment for each service is the lesser of the providers' charge, the carrier's fee schedule amount, or a national limit, set at 74 percent of the median of all carrier-fee-schedule amounts for each service. In practice, most lab claims are paid at the national limitation amounts. Clinical lab services in 2006 constituted slightly less than 2 percent of Medicare's spending. In that year, Medicare paid independent labs and physician offices $3.7 billion, and hospitals $3.2 billion for laboratory testing. Hospital-based labs' share of total clinical lab spending increased from 34 percent in 1996 to 46 percent in 2006. MedPAC, *A Data Book* (2007), p. 194.

52. For durable medical equipment (DME), Medicare pays the lesser of the provider's charge and a state fee schedule amount, initially calculated from allowed charges in 1986 and subsequently adjusted for inflation. Standard Part B cost sharing applies. In a 2000–02 demonstration, competitive bidding lowered prices for selected DME items 17–22 percent. Analyses of the demonstration did not find serious quality or access issues. A competitive bidding process for DME will be phased in nationwide, starting with ten metropolitan statistical areas in 2008 and expanding to eighty areas by 2009. Medicare payments accounted for 30 percent of retail expenditures on durable medical equipment in 2007 and

are expected to increase to 39 percent by 2017. MedPAC, *Medicare Payment Basics: Durable Medical Equipment Payment System* (October 2007). CMS, National Health Expenditure Projections (www.cms.hhs.gov/NationalHealthExpendData). Medicare pays dialysis facilities a predetermined payment for each dialysis treatment they furnish, using a prospective payment system first implemented in 1983. Providers separately bill Medicare for certain injectable medications, and in 2006 drugs accounted for about 35 percent of facilities' Medicare payments. Standard Part B cost sharing applies for both composite rate services and separately billable drugs. Medicare spending for dialysis and dialysis-related drugs totaled $8.4 billion in 2006 (or about 2 percent of total Medicare spending), an increase of 6 percent compared with 2005. Medicare expenditures for composite rate services and separately billable dialysis drugs averaged about $26,000 per patient in 2006. MedPAC, *Medicare Payment Basics: Outpatient Dialysis Services Payment System* (October 2007). MedPAC, *Report to Congress: Medicare Payment Policy* (2008), p. 113.

53. FFS spending on dialysis, clinical lab work, durable medical equipment, ambulance service, ambulatory surgical centers, rural health clinics, federally qualified health centers, outpatient rehabilitation facilities, and physician-administered drugs totaled 10 percent of Medicare outlays in 2007. FHI Board of Trustees, *2008 Annual Report*, table IV.B7.

54. In 2006, 44 percent of the elderly reported taking 3–6 prescription drugs, and 24 percent reported taking 7 or more. Seniors filled 4.9 prescriptions for drugs on average in that year, the figure rising to 6.3 for seniors with three or more chronic conditions. Kaiser Family Foundation, "Medicare Prescription Drug Benefit Progress Report: Findings from the Kaiser/Commonwealth/Tufts–New England Medical Center 2006 National Survey of Seniors and Prescription Drugs" (Menlo Park, Calif., August 2007) (www.kff.org/medicare/upload/7687.pdf). Estimated prescription drug expenditures by the elderly totaled $81.0 billion in 2007, about 35 percent of total prescription drug spending in that year. Authors' calculations based on CMS National Health Care Expenditure Projections and Age Estimates (www.cms.hhs.gov/NationalHealthExpendData).

55. In 2003, 29 percent of seniors obtained drug coverage through an employer-sponsored retiree policy, 9 percent through an HMO, 20 percent through Medigap or other private source, 9 percent through Medicaid or a state pharmaceutical assistance plan, and 6 percent through the Veterans Health Administration or other public source; 27 percent had no coverage. Dana Safran and others, "Prescription Drug Coverage and Seniors: Findings from a 2003 National Survey," *Health Affairs*, Web Exclusive (April 19, 2005): W152–66.

56. As of late 2005, only 6.3 million people—less than 15 percent of all Medicare beneficiaries—had enrolled in the discount card program. More than 1.8 million of these individuals received transitional assistance. The program was designed as a stopgap measure, to provide assistance to Medicare beneficiaries for the nineteen months before the implementation of Part D. Beneficiaries were charged up to $30 a year for the card, which gave them access to at least one drug in each of 209 therapeutic classes. Those with incomes below 135 percent of the poverty threshold did not have to pay the annual fee, had access to an annual credit of $600 to cover drug expenditures, and when this credit was exhausted paid only a fraction of the cost. Those with incomes below the poverty threshold paid 5 percent coinsurance, and those with incomes between 100 and 135 percent of the poverty threshold paid 10 percent. CMS analysis in early 2006 showed that beneficiaries in these categories could obtain discounts of 12–21 percent and 45–75 percent, respectively, on

commonly used brand-name and generic drugs. The CMS also found that limited-income beneficiaries could save much more, almost 44–92 percent over national average retail pharmacy prices, when using the card with the best prices and the $600 in transitional assistance. These savings were confirmed in independent analyses by the Lewin Group, American Enterprise Institute, and Kaiser Family Foundation. Using various methodologies, Lewin found a discount of more than 20 percent. Kaiser found 8–61 percent savings depending on the specific drug, card program, and pharmacy location. And AEI found limited-income seniors can save half to three-quarters of drug costs with the card in comparison with other private alternatives. CMS, *Evaluation of the Medicare-Approved Prescription Drug Discount Card and Transitional Assistance Program* (Abt Associates, May 2006), pp. A1–2 (www.cms.hhs.gov/reports/downloads/hassol.pdf).

57. A beneficiary cannot obtain drug coverage through a stand-alone plan if he or she receives benefits from a Medicare Advantage plan.

58. This includes enhanced plans. The 2008 monthly PDP premium excluding enhanced plans was $30.14. In 2008 all nonterritory beneficiaries had access to at least one PDP with monthly premiums of less than $18. The average of the lowest-cost PDP in each region was $14.98. Premiums ranged from $9.80 for the cheapest defined standard plan to $72 and $107.50 for the costliest basic and enhanced plan, respectively. Authors' calculation based on CMS, "2008 PDP Landscape Source" (www.cms.hhs.gov/PrescriptionDrugCov GenIn).

59. Benefit thresholds for the standard benefit will increase with the growth of per capita Medicare drug spending. For 2008 plans, cost sharing in the catastrophic range is the greater of 5 percent or $2.25 for generic and preferred formulary drugs and $5.60 for all other drugs.

60. Insurers have the option of offering defined standard coverage with different, actuarially equivalent cost sharing such as tiered co-payments of a low dollar amount for generic drugs and higher amounts for brand drugs in lieu of the standard 25 percent coinsurance. All other benefit design elements of these "actuarially equivalent standard" plans remain the same. Insurers may also offer "basic alternative" plans with the same actuarial value as the defined standard coverage, although with a reduced or eliminated deductible in addition to tiered cost sharing. Insurers may also offer "enhanced alternative" plans with actuarial values greater than the defined standard coverage. These plans can reduce or eliminate the deductible or initial coverage limit and also offer coverage for drugs in the doughnut hole. Since cost sharing under these plans is reduced in relation to the standard benefit, the threshold for catastrophic coverage effectively increases in total drug expenditures while the out-of-pocket threshold remains at $4,050. However, the beneficiary is responsible for the additional cost that exceeds the defined standard coverage, typically through higher premiums. Plan sponsors must include one basic plan (defined standard, actuarially equivalent, or basic alternative) among their offerings in each region. Twelve percent of all plans offered in 2008 were the standard benefit, 13 percent were actuarially equivalent standard, 25 percent were basic alternative, and 51 percent were enhanced alternative.

61. The two-drug requirement does not apply when only one drug is available for a particular category or class, or when only two drugs are available and one is clinically superior to the other. The formulary must not be designed to dissuade high-risk individuals, a test that can be met if the plan uses the model formulary of pharmacological classes designed for Medicare by the U.S. Pharmacopeia. Version 3.0 (for 2008 plans) had 138 unique classes.

To further dampen plans' incentive to enroll healthy people, CMS requires "all or substantially all" of the drugs in the antidepressant, antipsychotic, anticonvulsant, antineoplastic, immunosuppressant, and antiretroviral categories to be included. "Substantially all" means that all drugs in the protected classes are expected to be included in plan formularies, with the exceptions of multisource brands of identical molecular structure, extended release products when an immediate-release product is included, products that have the same active ingredient, and dosage forms that do not provide a unique route of administration (such as tablets and capsules). CMS also did not permit plans to employ techniques to manage use on beneficiaries stabilized on a drug regimen in one or more of these six categories before the introduction of Part D, unless they could demonstrate extraordinary circumstances. Plans may use techniques to manage therapy beneficiaries who *begin* treatment with drugs in these categories other than HIV/AIDS drugs.

62. The one exception is state pharmaceutical assistance plans. The catastrophic threshold is statutorily defined as $4,050 in out-of-pocket expenditures, which under the basic structure occurs when total expenditures on drugs reach $5,726.25.

63. See chapter 1 for a description of the design and political fate of the Medicare Catastrophic Coverage Act of 1988.

64. Sticks were also employed to encourage early enrollment of healthy people. In particular, Part D imposes a permanent increase in premiums for those who enroll late: for each month after which enrollees are eligible for Part D but do not sign up, they pay an additional 1 percent of the national base beneficiary premium ($27.93 in 2008) for their chosen plan. In other words, two years of delay costs enrollees an additional 24 percent of the national base beneficiary premium for every subsequent month in which they enroll in the program. It is easy to see that the cost of a PDP premium could be substantially larger if a retired person waited until seventy before enrolling, rather than enrolling at sixty-five. This penalty may be part of the explanation for the popularity of low premium plans.

65. Plan sponsors are paid 28 percent of each beneficiary's gross drug costs between the deductible and a catastrophic cost limit ($275 and $5,600 in 2008). The Congressional Budget Office (CBO) estimated that in 2006 this subsidy would cost Medicare about two-thirds as much as it would if the sponsor dropped coverage and participants joined a PDP.

66. MedPAC, *A Data Book* (2007), p. 61.

67. The proportion of employers with 500 or more employees providing supplementary coverage to Medicare-eligible retirees fell from 40 percent in 1993 to 21 percent in 2005. Mercer, "National Survey of Employer-Sponsored Health Plans" (2005).

68. Each provides core benefits, including 365 days of hospital coverage after patients have used up the standard Medicare coverage; coverage for Part A, Part B, and preventative care coinsurance; and up to three pints of blood a year. The most basic Medigap plan (plan A) provides only these benefits. Others provide additional benefits. CMS and National Association of Insurance Commissioners, *2007 Choosing a Medigap Policy: A Guide to Health Insurance for People with Medicare*, Publication 02110 (March 2007). Three states that had reformed their supplemental insurance market before the federal legislation was passed—Massachusetts, Minnesota, and Wisconsin—were permitted to offer plans with different combinations of benefits. Also, beneficiaries with policies issued before 1992 were allowed to continue them. These two types of nonstandard policies make up about 35 percent of all Medigap policies, but their numbers should fall rapidly as beneficiaries with the preexisting policies die.

69. Community-rated premiums are the same for all purchasers in a given area. Attained-age premiums differ according to the current age of the purchaser. Issue-age premiums are the same for all those who first purchase at a given age. Premiums for most policies vary with the participant's age. Thus Medigap premiums increase substantially as beneficiaries age. The 1990 reforms did not require insurers to offer all plans or to sell plans throughout the nation, however. Premiums vary greatly from state to state and even between different insurers within states. For instance, Plan A premiums ranged from $355 to $6,723 in 2006, a nineteen-fold difference. Donna O'Rourke, "TheStreet.com Ratings: Medigap Plans Vary in Price," *The Street.com* (www.thestreet.com/newsanalysis/ratings/10308492.html?puc=_tscs [September 2006]).

70. Among noninstitutionalized fee-for-service beneficiaries. MedPAC, *A Data Book* (2007), p. 61.

71. Ibid., p. 62.

72. About half of the states limit Medicaid eligibility for the elderly to people with incomes at or below 74 percent of the federal poverty level—the income test for Supplemental Security Income benefits and the minimum that states must abide by in order to receive federal matching funds. Most of the remaining states provide Medicaid to the elderly with incomes at or below 100 percent of the poverty threshold. See Kaiser Commission on Medicaid and the Uninsured, *Medicaid: A Primer* (Menlo Park, Calif., March 2007); and Medicaid/SCHIP eligibility levels, renewal, and enrollment practices at www.statehealthfacts.org.

73. FHI Board of Trustees, *2007 Annual Report*, table III.A3, and *2005 Annual Report*, table III.A3.

74. Between 1999 and 2003, the fraction of MA enrollees that were charged no supplemental premium for their MA coverage fell from 80 percent to 38 percent, the fraction offered any drug coverage fell from 84 percent to 69 percent, and the fraction offered preventive dental benefits dropped from 70 percent to 19 percent. Over this period, the fraction facing a co-payment for inpatient hospital admission soared from 4 percent to 82 percent, and the fraction facing co-payments exceeding $5 for a primary care physician visit rose from 38 percent to 87 percent. Lori Achman and Marsha Gold, *Medicare+Choice Plans Continue to Shift More Costs to Enrollees* (New York: Commonwealth Fund, April 2003) (www.cmwf.org/programs/medfutur/achman_m+cshiftcosts_628.pdf).

75. Enrollment in all prepaid plans peaked at 7,029,203 in November 1999 and then sank to 5,292,265 in February 2004. From November 1999 to February 2004, prepaid plan enrollment dropped by 1.7 million, or 25 percent. Between 1998 and 2002, the number of prepaid plans fell by more than half. In December 1998, there were 456 contracts; in February 2002, there were only 224. CMS, Health Plans, Reports, Files and Data, Monthly Reports, 1985–2005 (www.cms.hhs.gov/HealthPlanRepFileData).

76. These bids are compared to county benchmarks. If a plan's bid is below the benchmark, Medicare pays the plan the bid amount, and enrollees receive 75 percent of the difference between the bid and benchmark. Enrollees have the option of using this rebate to reduce Part B and Part D premiums or to purchase extra benefits that their plan may offer. If the bid exceeds the benchmark, the plan is paid the benchmark amount, and enrollees are required to pay supplemental premiums equal to the difference between the bid and the benchmark. Under MMA's provisions, county benchmarks are updated annually in one of three ways—using whichever method results in the highest increased benchmark. First, the

local benchmarks may be updated by the national growth rate in per capita Medicare spending (the general practice). Second, if the national growth rate is less than 2 percent, benchmarks are increased by 2 percent. Third, the benchmark of a given county may be set at an amount equal to the FFS expenditure level for the county. For purposes of implementing the third provision, CMS is required to determine FFS rates for each county at least every three years.

77. The MA permits two additional local coordinated (managed) care plans (CCPs)—preferred provider organizations (PPOs) and provider-sponsored organizations (PSOs)—as well as regional PPOs, private fee-for-service plans (PFFS), HMO Cost plans that are reimbursed on a cost basis, catastrophic insurance combined with medical saving accounts, programs for all-inclusive care of the elderly (PACE), demonstration plans, and separate pilot programs such as the Medicare Health Support Pilot, which provides care management services for beneficiaries with chronic conditions. As of March 2008, there were 9 catastrophic plans with a combined enrollment of 3,328 (0.03 percent of the prepaid plan total), 17 demonstration plans enrolling 4,176 (0.04 percent), 48 PACE plans enrolling 14,006 (0.14 percent of the total), 4 PSOs enrolling 16,486 (0.17 percent), 13 pilot plans enrolling 86,826 (0.89 percent), 14 regional PPOs enrolling 261,962 (2.7 percent), 38 cost plans enrolling 346,014 (3.6 percent), 137 Local PPOs enrolling 578,795 (6 percent), 79 PFFS plans enrolling 2,108,721 (21.7 percent), and 368 HMOs enrolling 6,295,393 (64.8 percent). CMS, *Part D Enrollment Data, Monthly Enrollment by Contract* (March 2008).

78. PFFS plans accounted for a small share of total MA enrollment in 2008 (22 percent), but the rate of growth in enrollment far exceeds that for HMOs and PPOs between December 2005 and March 2008 (about 1.5 times). During this period, PFFS enrollment increased from nearly 209,000 to 2.1 million, or more than tenfold.

79. CMS, *Part D Enrollment Data.* MSAs are available in all fifty states and the District of Columbia, as well as Puerto Rico, Guam, and the U.S. Virgin Islands. Medicare makes an annual deposit into an interest-bearing account on behalf of enrollees, who may use these funds to pay for qualified health care expenses until they meet the deductible, at which point the plan will pay for all Medicare-covered services.

80. In March 2007, total SNP enrollment reached 1,130,264; the majority of enrollees were dual-eligibles (815,569). The number of SNPs rose from 125 to 477 between 2005 and 2007, and to 769 in 2008.

81. Regional PPOs must offer services throughout at least one of twenty-six regions, each of which covers, at a minimum, a single state. These PPOs were introduced in an effort to provide beneficiaries in rural areas greater access to MA plans. They offer a benefit package that has a single deductible (rather than the separate deductibles for Parts A and B) and provides catastrophic limits on out-of-pocket expenditures. The law does not specify the level of the single deductible or the catastrophic limit. As of March 2008, enrollment remains modest at about 262,000. The regional PPOs are paid through competitive bidding. Each PPO submits a single bid for an entire region. That bid is compared to a benchmark constructed as the average of all the local county benchmarks in the region, weighted by the Medicare population in each county, combined with the average of the regional PPO bids. The bid component of the final benchmark for each region is given a weight equal to the national level of MA penetration (the percent of Medicare beneficiaries enrolled in MA across the nation). To encourage the creation and continuity of regional PPOs, the MMA established a bonus pool that is distributed either uniformly to all regional plans or

as targeted payments to encourage plans to enter or remain in underserved regions. This bonus pool was initially equal to $10 billion plus one-half of the government's savings derived from bids by regional plans that fall below the benchmark over the 2007–13 period. The Tax Relief and Health Care Act of 2006 reduced the stabilization fund to $3.5 billion over five years to offset the cost of the 2007 freeze on the physician fee schedule conversion factor. The Medicare, Medicaid, and SCHIP Extension Act of 2007 provided for an additional drawdown of $1.5 billion in 2012. Congress has reduced the amount available in this pool primarily because a sufficient number of regional PPOs have emerged to participate in Medicare.

82. Some overpayments were much higher than this average: 117 percent for the large urban counties and 128 percent for rural counties. Payments also varied by plan type. PFFS plans have among the highest program payments in relation to FFS expenditures at 117 percent, reflecting their concentration in certain counties that have very high relative benchmark levels compared with other geographic areas. The main source of the variation by area reflects statutory provisions that introduced minimum county payment rates, or floors, intended to attract or retain private plans in counties paid at a floor rate. Floor rates as such are no longer a basis of plan payment, but what were historically floor counties generally continue to have higher payment rates than nonfloor counties in relation to FFS expenditure levels. Local PPOs have the highest program payments in relation to FFS, owing to concentration in floor counties and also less aggressive bidding on the part of such plans (reflecting the looser network structure and coverage of out-of-network care). The payment level for regional PPOs is the lowest among plan types because regional plans cannot select which counties to include in their service area (that is, they cannot choose to operate only in urban counties or only in rural counties) and because the formula used to determine regional benchmarks is population based. MedPAC, *Medicare Payment Policy* (2008), pp. 246–47.

83. Medicare actuaries project exhaustion of the HI trust fund in early 2019. FHI Board of Trustees, *2008 Annual Report*, p. 15; CBO, *Reducing the Deficit: Spending and Revenue Options* (February 2007); Richard Foster, "The Financial Outlook for Medicare," Testimony before the House Subcommittee on Health, Committee on Ways and Means, 110 Cong. 2 sess. (GPO, April 1, 2008) (http://waysandmeans.house.gov/media/pdf/110/RSFTestimony.pdf).

84. FHI Board of Trustees, *2008 Annual Report*, table III.A3. The number of MA plans nearly tripled from February 2004 to March 2008. Local CCPs and PFFS plans accounted for 52 percent and 47 percent of the enrollment growth over this period, respectively. CMS, Health Plans, Reports, Files and Data, Monthly Reports, 1985–2005 (www.cms.hhs.gov/HealthPlanRepFileData); CMS, Medicare Advantage/Part D Contract and Enrollment Data, Monthly Contract and Enrollment Summary Report (www.cms.hhs.gov/MCRAdvPartDEnrolData).

85. In 2008, 85 percent could enroll in a local HMO or PPO, 87 percent in a regional PPO, and 100 percent in MSAs or PFFS plans. MedPAC, *Report to the Congress: Medicare Payment Policy* (2008), p. 245.

86. FHI Board of Trustees, *2008 Annual Report*, table III.A3. The CBO agrees and expects MA enrollment to equal 26 percent. In 2007 the House of Representatives passed legislation to eliminate the payment differential between traditional Medicare and MA. It is opposed by some in the Senate and is likely to continue to be the subject of debate.

87. FHI Board of Trustees, *2008 Annual Report*, table III.A4.

88. The other sources of income include payments from the railroad retirement system, general revenues to pay for benefits for a small number of uninsured people and for some former military personnel, and premiums from voluntary enrollees who are otherwise not entitled to benefits.

89. These reserves must be invested exclusively in securities guaranteed as to principal and interest by the U.S. government.

90. The SMI trust fund maintains only a contingency reserve, which historically has been set at about 28 percent of excess of assets over liabilities to the following year's total incurred expenditures. Past studies have indicated that a ratio of roughly 15–20 percent is sufficient to protect against unforeseen contingencies. At the end of 2007, the Part B reserve ratio was 22 percent, or slightly above normal requirements—the first occurrence of a fully adequate Part B contingency reserve since 2002. FHI Board of Trustees, *2008 Annual Report*, p. 103.

91. Ibid., p. 15.

92. The Board of Trustees issued a third consecutive determination of projected "excess general revenue Medicare funding" in its 2008 report. In February 2008 President Bush submitted legislation responding to the "Medicare funding warning" triggered by the 2007 Medicare Trustees Report. As required by law, the president must again submit to Congress proposed legislation to respond to the warning, and Congress must consider the legislation on an expedited basis.

93. The gap is 62 percent versus 51 percent. Karen Davis and others, "Medicare vs. Private Insurance: Rhetoric and Reality," *Health Affairs*, Web Exclusive (October 9, 2002): W311–24.

# Chapter 3

1. Only 1.5 percent of the elderly, compared with 20.2 percent of nonelderly adults, were without health insurance during 2006. U.S. Bureau of the Census, *Current Population Survey,* Annual Social and Economic Supplement (March 2007) (http://pubdb3.census.gov/macro/032007/health/h01_001.htm).

2. In 2008 the Medicare actuaries projected HI expenditures to exceed total income in 2010 and later, requiring redemption of trust fund assets to cover the difference. The HI trust fund assets are projected to be exhausted in early 2019. Federal Hospital Insurance (FHI) Board of Trustees, *2008 Annual Report of the Board of Trustees of the Federal Hospital Insurance and Federal Supplementary Medical Insurance Trust Funds* (2008), p. 15.

3. Henry J. Aaron, "Budget Crisis, Entitlement Crisis, Health Care Financing Problem—Which Is It?" *Health Affairs* 26 (November/December 2007): 1622–33.

4. Roughly one in ten elderly visits to physicians are well visits. Janet Heinrich, "Medicare Preventive Services," Hearings before the House Subcommittee on Health, Committee on Energy and Commerce, GAO-04-1004T (U.S. Government Accountability Office, September 21, 2004) (www.gao.gov/new.items/d041004t.pdf). About 18 percent of people aged seventy or older report trouble with their eyesight and a third report problems with hearing. V. A. Campbell and others, "Surveillance for Sensory Impairment, Activity Limitation, and Health-Related Quality of Life among Older Adults: Surveillance for

Selected Public Health Indicators Affecting Older Adults—United States, 1993–1997," *MMWR CDC Surveillance Summary* 48(8) (1999): 131–56.

5. In 2006 the overall coinsurance rate for hospital outpatient services was about 33 percent. The coinsurance rate is different for each service. Some services, such as imaging, have very high rates of coinsurance—42 percent. Other services, such as evaluation and management, have coinsurance rates of 23 percent. Historically, beneficiary coinsurance payments for hospital outpatient services were based on hospital charges, while Medicare payments were based on hospital costs. As hospital charges grew faster than costs, coinsurance represented a large share of total payment over time. In adopting the outpatient prospective payment system, Congress froze the dollar amounts for coinsurance. Consequently, beneficiaries' share of total payments will decline over time but CMS has estimated that it could take three to four decades before the coinsurance for all procedures reaches 20 percent. MedPAC, *A Data Book: Healthcare Spending and the Medicare Program* (June 2007), pp. 109, 113.

6. The 2007 inpatient hospital deductible was $992, compared with an average deductible of $323 for HMOs and $334 for PPOs among workers with a separate hospital deductible in 2007. Kaiser Family Foundation, *Employer Health Benefits 2007* (Menlo Park, Calif., September 2007), p. 103.

7. In 2007 the average coinsurance rate for outpatient surgery and primary care physician office visits in employer-sponsored plans was 18 percent and 17 percent, respectively. Ibid., pp. 105, 107.

8. Ibid., p. 111. As an exception to the rule, regional preferred provider organizations and medical savings account plans under Medicare Advantage are required to have benefit structures that include an out-of-pocket limit on enrollee expenditures. The plans are allowed to determine their own level of out-of-pocket limits.

9. MedPAC, *A Data Book* (2007), pp. 51–52. Clearly, whether and what type of supplemental coverage beneficiaries have affects their ability to obtain care. In 2003 about 19 percent of Medicare beneficiaries with no supplemental coverage reported delaying care because of cost, compared with about 5 percent of those with retiree or Medigap coverage. Medicare Current Beneficiary Survey data tables (www.cms.hhs.gov/MCBS/Downloads/CNP_2003_section5.pdf).

10. Most physicians—almost 97 percent—accept at least some new fee-for-service Medicare patients, and a smaller share—80 percent—accept all or most. The number of physicians providing services to beneficiaries has more than kept pace with growth in the beneficiary population. From 2001 to 2006, the number of physicians who billed Medicare grew faster than Medicare Part B enrollment. During this time, Part B enrollment grew 6.9 percent. By comparison, the number of physicians with 15 or more Medicare patients grew 8.7 percent. The number of physicians with 200 or more Medicare patients grew even faster, at 12.9 percent. Overall, the number of physicians per 1,000 beneficiaries has remained steady at about 14. MedPAC, *Report to the Congress: Medicare Payment Policy* (March 2008), pp. 87–88.

11. In addition, between 2005 and 2007, aged beneficiaries consistently reported higher levels of satisfaction with the timeliness of health care (for both routine care and illness or injury) compared with the near-elderly privately insured (aged fifty to sixty-four). Beneficiaries with disabilities are twice as likely as seniors to report problems with getting

needed care. MedPAC, *A Data Book* (2007), pp. 51, 56; and MedPAC, *Report to the Congress: Medicare Payment Policy* (2008), p. 88.

12. Early in the twentieth century a Boston surgeon published the results of what happened to surgical patients during the five years following hospital discharge, including avoidable errors. For his trouble, he was nearly expelled from the Massachusetts Medical Society. T. Andrew Dodds, "Richard Cabot: Medical Reformer during the Progressive Era (1890–1920)," *Annals of Internal Medicine* 119 (September 1993): 417–22.

13. Martin Sipkoff, "The New Consensus Favoring IOM's Definition of Quality," *Managed Care Magazine,* June 2004 (www.managedcaremag.com/archives/0406/0406.quality_defined.html).

14. Mark R. Chassin, "Is Health Care Ready for Six Sigma Quality?" *Milbank Quarterly* 76 (December 1998): 565–91. Overuse includes the excessive prescription of tranquilizers or sedatives. Underuse includes the failure to prescribe beta-blockers and low-dose aspirin to patients who have suffered heart attacks. Misuse includes giving incorrect dosages and prescribing the wrong medications.

15. Elizabeth A. McGlynn and others, "The Quality of Health Care Delivered to Adults in the United States," *New England Journal of Medicine* 348 (June 2003): 2635–45.

16. Appropriate timing of antibiotics includes receiving prophylactic antibiotics within one hour prior to surgical incision and discontinuing the antibiotics within twenty-four hours after surgery ends. Agency for Healthcare Research and Quality, *National Health Care Quality Report, 2006* (Rockville, Md., 2006).

17. The vast majority of adverse drug events in 2004 (90.3 percent, or 1,093,600 hospital stays) represented adverse effects of properly administered drugs (in terms of dosage). These consisted of adverse reactions, including allergic or hypersensitivity reactions, caused by drugs properly administered in therapeutic and prophylactic dosages. Most remaining adverse drug events (8.6 percent, or 104,200 stays) were drug poisoning (which involve accidental drug overdose), wrong drugs taken or given in error, or drugs taken inadvertently. The remaining 1.1 percent of coded adverse drug events include neuropathy or dermatitis due to drugs. Anne Elixhauser and Pamela Owens, "Adverse Drug Events in U.S. Hospitals, 2004," Healthcare Cost and Utilization Project Statistical Brief 29 (Rockville, Md.: Agency for Healthcare Research and Quality, April 2007).

18. MedPAC, *Report to the Congress: Medicare Payment Policy* (2008), pp. 53–54.

19. Cathy Schoen and others, "Taking the Pulse of Health Care Systems: Experiences of Patients with Health Problems in Six Countries," *Health Affairs,* Web Exclusive (November 3, 2005): W509–25.

20. Jean Abraham, Roger Feldman, and Caroline Carlin, "Understanding Employee Awareness of Health Care Quality Information: How Can Employers Benefit?" *Health Services Research* (December 2004).

21. The NCQA's HEDIS instrument measures many dimensions of performance, such as the percentage of women aged fifty-two to sixty-nine who received a mammogram within the past two years and the percentage of adult women who received a Pap test within the past three years. See www.ncqa.org/tabid/59/Default.aspx.

22. Social Security Act amendments of 1965, P.L. 89-97, sec. 1801.

23. Institute of Medicine, *Medicare: A Strategy for Quality Assurance*, vol. 1 (Washington: National Academy of Sciences, 1990), pp. 139–206.

24. Institute of Medicine, *Pathways to Quality Health Care: Medicare's Quality Improvement Organization Program: Maximizing Potential* (Washington: National Academy of Sciences, 2006).

25. Thomas Lee, James Mongan, and Robert Mechanic, "Transforming U.S. Health Care: Policy Challenges Affecting the Integration and Improvement of Care," Health Policy Issues and Options Series, 2006-01 (Brookings, 2006); Thomas Lee and James Mongan, "Are Healthcare's Problems Incurable? One Integrated Delivery System's Program for Transforming Its Care," Health Policy Issues and Options Series, 2006-02 (Brookings, 2006).

26. See CMS, Office of Public Affairs, "Medicare 'Pay for Performance (P4P)' Initiatives," Press Release, January 31, 2005 (www.cms.hhs.gov/apps/media/press/release.asp?Counter=1343).

27. Social Security Act amendments of 1965, P.L. 89-97, sec. 1862 (a)(1)(A). This phrase was put in the act at the last minute, lifted from an Aetna policy available to federal employees in 1965. The relevant passage in the Aetna policy is in the section entitled "Exclusions" and states: "Charges listed on this and the following page are not allowable: Charges for services and supplies . . . not *reasonably necessary* for treatment of pregnancy, illness, or injury, or to improve the functioning of a malformed body member." Notably, for Aetna and other insurance companies (including the Blue Cross and Blue Shield plans) operating at that time, "reasonably necessary" was not an effective cost-saving feature of health plans and was not used as one. For an unofficial history of the phrase, see Jacqueline Fox, "Medicare Should, but Cannot, Consider Costs: Legal Impediments to a Sound Policy," *Buffalo Law Review* 53 (Spring 2005): 577–633.

28. CMS staff, an independent contractor, or the Medicare Coverage Advisory Committee may conduct these studies. Once a coverage decision has been made, a code and payment rate must be provided and instructions disseminated to contractors. The entire process can take anywhere from a few months to several years. Private insurers often approve payment for devices, biologicals, or procedures long before Medicare does. For example, private plans covered kidney transplants many years before Medicare did in 1973. Hospitals offered implantable defibrillators to private patients several years before Medicare paid for these devices. Medicare did not pay for diagnostic PET scans for a wide variety of cancers until 2002, although such tests had been covered by many private insurers for the better part of a decade. The Medicare, Medicaid, and SCHIP Benefits Improvement Act of 2000 requires the secretary of the Department of Health and Human Services (HHS) to report annually to Congress on the length of time it takes to make national coverage decisions. See Tommy G. Thompson, HHS secretary, *Report to Congress on National Coverage Decisions* (June 4, 2002).

29. As a result of the Medicare Modernization Act of 2003, timelines for processing national coverage determinations (NCDs) were shortened to six months for most NCDs not requiring technology assessment and nine months for those with technology assessment. Barry M. Straube, "How Changes in the Medicare Coverage Process Have Facilitated the Spread of New Technologies," *Health Affairs*, Web Exclusive (June 23, 2005): W314–16.

30. At least forty-five health technology assessment (HTA) agencies currently exist in twenty-three countries. Nearly every European country has an HTA agency that is also a member of the Health Evidence Network of the European bloc of the World Health

Organization. Notably, Japan—the world's second largest health care market—like the United States, also lacks a national agency devoted to health technology appraisals. See Corinna Sorenson, Michael Drummond, and Panos Kanavos, *Ensuring Value for Money in Health Care: The Role of Health Technology Assessment in the European Union* (London: European Observatory on Health Systems and Policies, April 2008); Health Evidence Network of the European Regional Office of the World Health Organization (www.euro.who.int/HEN); and International Network of Agencies for Health Technology Assessment (www.inahta.org/Members).

31. Failed U.S. HTA agencies that have advised HCFA/CMS include the Health Program of the Congressional Office of Technology Assessment, 1972–95; National Center for Health Care Technology, 1978–81; Office of Health Technology Assessment, 1981–95; Council on Health Care Technology, 1984–89. John Eisenberg and Deborah Zarin, "Health Technology Assessment in the United States: Past, Present, and Future," *International Journal of Technology Assessment in Health Care* 18 (May 2002): 192–98. However, renewed interest emerged in 2007, when the House of Representatives passed a bill calling for a new center for comparative effectiveness, funded by public and private payers.

32. Karen Davis and others, "Medicare Versus Private Insurance: Rhetoric and Reality," *Health Affairs*, Web Exclusive (October 9, 2002): W311–24.

33. Patients rate highly providers who communicate well with them. But communicative physicians were not found to deliver technically better care, on the average, than do their more taciturn colleagues. Satisfied patients may still have better health outcomes because they are more willing than unsatisfied patients to take medications and follow advice. John T. Chang and others, "Patients' Global Ratings of Their Health Care Are Not Associated with the Technical Quality of Their Care," *Annals of Internal Medicine* 144 (May 2006): 665–72. In 2003 the proportion of seniors who reported that their health care provider sometimes or never listened carefully to them, explained things clearly, showed respect for what they had to say, and spent enough time with them was 6.3 percent, nearly three-fifths the rate for people aged eighteen to sixty-four. Agency for Healthcare Research and Quality, *National Health Care Quality Report, 2006.*

34. Calculated from data in FHI Board of Trustees, *2008 Annual Report*; Bureau of Economic Analysis, "Current-Dollar and 'Real' Gross Domestic Product" (March 27, 2008); and U.S. Bureau of the Census, *Statistical Abstract of the United States: 2008* (2008).

35. Congressional Budget Office (CBO), *The Long-Term Outlook for Health Care Spending* (November 2007).

36. According to the Medicare trustees, "Over long historical periods, average, demographically adjusted, per capita growth rates have been similar for Medicare and private health insurance." From 1975 to 2005, real spending per beneficiary in Medicare increased at an average rate of 4.6 percent, compared with an average real per capita growth rate of 4.1 percent for private insurers. From 1990 to 2005, these figures were 3.8 percent and 3.1 percent, respectively. FHI Board of Trustees, *2008 Annual Report*, p. 41; CBO, *The Long-Term Outlook for Health Care Spending*, table 2.

37. In the early to mid-1990s, Medicare rates were about two-thirds of commercial payment rates for physician services, but since 1999 Medicare rates have consistently been in the neighborhood of 80 percent of commercial rates. Enrollment shifts in the private market from higher-paying indemnity plans to lower-paying health maintenance organizations accounted for much of the narrowing between Medicare and private insurance rates from

the mid-1990s to 2001. Averaged across all services and areas, 2006 Medicare rates were 81.3 percent of extrapolated private rates, compared with 82.6 percent in 2005. MedPAC, *Medicare Payment Policy* (2008), p. 89.

38. See CMS, National Health Expenditure Data (www.cms.hhs.gov/NationalHealth ExpendData); Mark E. Litow, "Medicare versus Private Health Insurance: The Cost of Administration" (Milwaukee, Wisc.: Milliman Inc.: January, 6, 2006) (www.cahi.org/cahi_contents/resources/pdf/CAHIMedicareTechnicalPaper.pdf); and Steffie Woolhandler and others, "Costs of Health Care Administration in the United States and Canada," *New England Journal of Medicine* 349 (August 2003): 768–75.

39. No component of GDP can permanently grow faster than the total. In a 2007 report, the CBO projected an eventual slowdown, starting in 2019, but occurring very gradually. CBO, *The Long-Term Outlook for Health Care Spending*.

40. According to the CBO, the pure effect of aging accounts for about one-quarter of the projected growth in federal Medicare and Medicaid spending through 2030. By 2050, that share falls to under 20 percent, and by 2082, to only about 10 percent. Ibid.

41. U.S. Department of Health and Human Services and Department of Justice. *Health Care Fraud and Abuse Control Program, Annual Report, FY 2006* (November 2007) (http://oig.hhs.gov/publications/docs/hcfac/hcfacreport2006.pdf).

42. Between 2001 and 2006, the volume of physician services per fee-for-service beneficiary grew at an average annual rate of 5.2 percent. Imaging and tests grew the most, at 9.1 and 6.9 percent, respectively. Overall volume increases translate directly to growth in Part B spending and are largely responsible for the negative updates required by the SGR formula. MedPAC, *Medicare Payment Policy* (2008), p. 93.

43. *The Dartmouth Atlas of Health Care,* Data Tables (www.dartmouthatlas.org). For a detailed discussion of the issue, see CBO, *Geographic Variation of Health Care Spending* (February 2008).

44. The five health regions with the lowest rates of hospital admissions for broken hips in 2003 averaged 5.01 per thousand Medicare enrollees, compared with 10.4 in the five health regions with highest rates, a ratio of just over two to one. By comparison, the five communities with lowest rates of admission for back surgery averaged 1.7 per thousand, while the five communities with highest rates averaged 8.82, a ratio of more than five to one. The five communities with the lowest rate of coronary catheterization averaged 4.8 per thousand, while the five highest averaged 28.7 per thousand, a ratio of six to one. And the highest region, Elyria, Ohio, had a rate of 42 per thousand. See *The Dartmouth Atlas of Health Care*, Tools (www.dartmouthatlas.org).

45. Jonathan S. Skinner, Douglas O. Staiger, and Elliott S. Fisher, "Is Technological Change in Medicine Always Worth It? The Case of Acute Myocardial Infarction," *Health Affairs*, Web Exclusive (February 7, 2006): W34–47.

46. In January 2002 CMS selected fifteen sites for a four-year pilot project (the Medicare Coordinated Care Demonstration) to test whether providing coordinated care services to Medicare fee-for-service beneficiaries with complex chronic conditions can yield better patient outcomes without increasing program costs. The selected projects represent a wide range of programs, use both case and disease management approaches, and operate in both urban and rural settings. The sites began implementing the project in April 2002. By September 2002, all fifteen sites had initiated enrollment. In 2006 eleven of the sites were extended for an additional two years to allow time for further data analyses. The

remaining four sites terminated operations as scheduled. One transferred to another Medicare demonstration, and the other three had insufficient enrollment to warrant continuation. In December 2007 the CMS completed the final review of the four-year evaluation data. While all of the sites appeared to have improved some aspects of quality of care, none showed a cost savings, and only three of the eleven operating sites showed a potential for budget neutrality. Overall, the demonstration increased Medicare spending for participating beneficiaries by about 11 percent, or approximately $16 million annually. Based on these results, the CMS extended the three potentially budget neutral sites for two more years to allow further study of their programs, contingent on their acceptance of fees reduced as needed to achieve budget neutrality. The remaining eight sites terminated operations as scheduled in 2008. CMS, *Medicare Coordinated Care Demonstration Fact Sheet* (December 2007) (www.cms.hhs.gov/DemoProjectsEvalRpts/downloads/CC_Fact_Sheet.pdf).

47. The two sites are Polk County, Florida, and San Antonio, Texas. U.S. Department of Health and Human Services, *Final Report to Congress: Evaluation of Medicare's Competitive Bidding Demonstration for Durable Medical Equipment, Prosthetics, Orthotics, and Supplies* (2004) (www.cms.hhs.gov/DemoProjectsEvalRpts/downloads/CMS_rtc.pdf).

48. Between 2002 and 2003, physicians in some health care markets received commercial payment rates for privately insured patients that went as high as 125 to 200 percent of the Medicare fee schedule. Sally Trude and Paul B. Ginsburg, "An Update on Medicare Beneficiary Access to Physician Services," Issue Brief 93 (Washington: Center for Studying Health System Change, February 2005).

49. Research published by the Center for Studying Health System Change (ibid.) has compared access rates by geographic area, with particular attention to the difference between Medicare and private insurer fees in each area. This research found that, despite differences in Medicare and commercial payment rates across markets, the proportion of Medicare beneficiaries reporting problems with access to care in markets with the widest payment rate gaps did not vary significantly from the proportion reporting problems in markets with more comparable payment rates. In addition, privately insured people aged fifty to sixty-four did not appear to gain better access to care in comparison with Medicare beneficiaries in markets with higher commercial payment rates. The unwillingness of providers to deny access to beneficiaries in areas with wide public-private payment differentials could be indicative of Medicare's dominant market power. MedPAC, *Medicare Payment Policy* (2008), pp. 85–86.

50. The exception is very high earners. Since 1986, the 2.9 percentage point hospital insurance tax levied divided equally between workers and employers applies to all earnings.

51. FHI Board of Trustees, *2008 Annual Report*, table III.A2. For the first ten years of the seventy-five-year projection period, short-range projections of Medicare costs are made separately for each category of health spending (for example, inpatient hospital, physician, and home health care) and are built up from assumptions about general price inflation, excess medical inflation for each category of spending, changes in utilization of services, and changes in the "intensity" or average complexity of services. Excess cost growth rates for years eleven through twenty-four are computed as smooth transitions from the excess growth rates for Medicare Parts A, B, and D in year ten of the projection period to the excess cost growth rate common to all parts of the Medicare program that is shown in year twenty-five (1.3 percent in 2032 for the 2008 FHI Trustees report). For the next fifty-one

years of the seventy-five-year period, the CMS actuaries assume that the annual growth of Medicare spending will exceed GDP growth by an average of 1 percentage point a year, eventually reaching close to 0 percent in the terminal year. Revenue projections are based on anticipated growth of taxable payroll and income taxes. Earmarked payroll and income taxes and other dedicated revenues are expected to increase negligibly as a share of GDP. For details on projection methods, see Todd Caldis, "The Long-Term Projection Assumptions for Medicare and Aggregate National Health Expenditures" (Washington: CMS, Office of the Actuary, March 25, 2008) (www.cms.hhs.gov/ReportsTrustFunds/downloads/projectionmethodology.pdf).

52. One way to gauge Medicare's financial condition is to view it from a unified federal budget perspective. In particular, this assessment determines whether Medicare receipts from the public (such as payroll taxes and beneficiary premiums) exceed or fall short of outlays to the public. Under this approach, interest income on the HI trust fund assets and contributions from general revenues to the SMI program are ignored, because they are essentially intragovernmental transfers between the general fund and the Medicare trust funds. As a result, the difference between public receipts and public expenditures for Medicare reflects any HI income shortfall and the general revenue share of SMI. American Academy of Actuaries, "Medicare's Financial Condition: Beyond Actuarial Balance," Issue Brief (April 2007) (www.actuary.org/pdf/medicare/trustees_07.pdf).

53. CBO, *The Long-Term Budget Outlook* (December 2007).

54. Rapid technological advance almost always leads to increased total spending on its new products. Official statistics indicate that health care prices have risen faster than other prices. But these statistics are seriously flawed. Careful studies of the price of particular medical treatments, including those for heart attacks and mental illness, show that if improvements in quality are measured more accurately than is done in computing official price indexes, the price of care has fallen. See Ernst R. Berndt and others, "Medical Care Prices and Output," in *Handbook of Health Economics*, vol. 1A, edited by Anthony Culyer and Joseph Newhouse (Amsterdam: Elsevier, 2000), pp. 119–80.

55. The measures in table 3-5 are predicated on the CBO assumption that, in the absence of major policy change, per capita health care spending will exceed income growth by 2.5 percentage points annually. In that event, additional general revenues equal to approximately 6.5 percent of GDP would be necessary.

56. Raising the age of eligibility from sixty-five to sixty-seven would reduce the number of beneficiaries by 9–10 percent between 2007 and 2050, but spending by only 3 percent. Raising the eligibility age to seventy would cut the rolls by more than 20 percent and spending by about 10 percent. CBO, *Budget Options* (February 2007), p. 166.

57. U.S. Social Security Administration, Office of Policy, *Annual Statistical Supplement, 2007* (2007) (www.ssa.gov/policy/docs/statcomps/supplement/2007/5a.html#table5.a3).

58. Richard W. Johnson, *Raising the Eligibility Age for Medicare: Can One Stone Kill Three Birds?* (Washington: Urban Institute, 2005) (www.urban.org/UploadedPDF/411253_medicare_eligibility.pdf).

59. The median income for adults aged sixty-five or older was $20,481 in 2004, with a distribution highly skewed toward the lower end. More than one-third of the elderly have incomes of less than $15,000. The majority (59 percent) have incomes of less than $25,000. Social Security Administration, *Income of the Aged Chartbook, 2004* (September 2006), p. 11.

60. Linqun Liu, Andrew J. Rettenmaier, and Zijun Wang, "The Rising Burden of Health Spending on Seniors" (Washington: National Center for Policy Analysis, February 2007).

61. As projected in CBO's ten-year baseline through 2017, then remains at the projected 2017 level as a share of GDP. CBO, *The Long-Term Budget Outlook*, p. 37.

## Chapter 4

1. E. J. Dionne, "Why Social Insurance?" Social Security Brief (Washington: National Academy of Social Insurance, January 6, 1999).

2. Ibid.

3. We draw ideas from numerous expert commissions, including the Medicare Payment Advisory Commission (MedPAC) and the National Academy of Social Insurance.

4. As in subsequent chapters on premium support and individual accounts, the model examined here is "purer" than could likely occur in reality. Our purpose is to emphasize each approach's differences and relative strengths and weaknesses. In chapter 7, we describe some hybrid plans that combine features from all three "pure" approaches.

5. See, for example, David A. Moss, *When All Else Fails: Government as the Ultimate Risk Manager* (Harvard University Press, 2004); Jacob S. Hacker, *The Great Risk Shift* (Oxford University Press, 2006).

6. Deborah Stone, "Social Insurance as Organized Altruism," presented at the National Academy of Social Insurance Conference (February 1, 2007).

7. *Public Papers of the Presidents of the United States: Lyndon B. Johnson, 1965*, vol. 2, entry 394 (Washington: GPO, 1966), pp. 811–15 (www.lbjlib.utexas.edu/johnson/archives.hom/speeches.hom/650730.asp).

8. John Halpin and Ruy Teixeira, "The Politics of Definition," *American Prospect*, April 20, 2006.

9. Arnold S. Relman, "Medicine and the Free Market: The Health of Nations," *New Republic*, March 7, 2005, pp. 22–30.

10. "Proposal of the Physicians' Working Group for Single-Payer National Health Insurance," *Journal of the American Medical Association* 290 (August 2003): 798–805.

11. James C. Robinson, "From Managed Care to Consumer Health Insurance: The Rise and Fall of Aetna," *Health Affairs* 23 (March/April 2004): 43–55.

12. Jonathan Oberlander, *The Political Life of Medicare* (University of Chicago Press, 2003).

13. Robert A. Berenson, "Doctoring Health Care II: Yo Democrats! Medicare Is Privatizing!" *American Prospect*, January 7, 2007; Jeanne Lambrew and Karen Davenport, "Has Medicare Been Privatized?" (Center for American Progress, February 8, 2006) (www.americanprogress.org/issues/2006/02/b1417251.html).

14. Representative Fortney (Pete) Stark, Statement, January 10, 2007 (www.house.gov/stark/news/110th/floorstatements/20070110_medicare.htm).

15. Rick Weiss, "A Tale of Politics: PET Scans' Change in Medicare Coverage," *Washington Post*, October 14, 2004, p. A1.

16. Since January 2005, the National Health Service has been legally obliged to fund medicines and treatments recommended by the technology appraisal board of the National Institute for Health and Clinical Excellence.

17. Alan Garber, "Cost-Effectiveness and Evidence Evaluation as Criteria for Coverage Policy," *Health Affairs*, Web Exclusive (May 19, 2004): W284–96. Blue Cross/Blue Shield use a Technology Evaluation Center to inform coverage policy.

18. For proposals for new initiatives in the United States, see Gail Wilensky, "Developing a Center for Comparative Effectiveness Information," *Health Affairs* 25, Web Exclusive (November/December 2006): W572–85. Ezekiel Emanuel, Victor Fuchs, and Alan Garber have suggested the creation of a federal agency with a budget exceeding $1 billion to carry out research to evaluate medical advances in "Essential Elements of a Technology and Outcomes Assessment Initiative," *Journal of the American Medical Association* 298 (September 2007): 1323–25. See also Wilhelmine Miller, *Value-Based Coverage Policy in the United States and the United Kingdom: Different Paths to a Common Goal*, Background Paper (Washington: National Health Policy Forum, November 29, 2006). For recommendations by MedPAC, see *Report to the Congress: Promoting Greater Efficiency in Medicare* (June 2007), pp. 27–54. For a discussion of an expanded federal role and implications for spending, see Congressional Budget Office (CBO), *Research on the Comparative Effectiveness of Medical Treatments: Issues and Options for an Expanded Federal Role* (December 2007). For a description of NICE, see www.nice.org.uk/ aboutNICE. For a description of benefits design in other countries, see Steven G. Morgan and others, "Centralized Drug Review Processes in Australia, Canada, New Zealand, and the United Kingdom," *Health Affairs* 25 (March/April 2006): 337–47. For U.S. experience, see, for example, Carolyn M. Clancy and Kelly Cronin, "Evidence-Based Decision Making: Global Evidence, Local Decisions," *Health Affairs* 24 (January/February 2005): 151–62; Ryan Padrez and others, *The Use of Oregon's Evidence-Based Reviews for Pharmacy Policies: Experiences in Four States* (Washington: Kaiser Commission for Medicaid and the Uninsured, May 2005).

19. Amitabh Chandra, Jonathan Gruber, and Robin McKnight, "Patient Cost-Sharing, Hospitalization Offsets, and the Design of Optimal Health Insurance for the Elderly," Working Paper 12972 (Cambridge, Mass.: National Bureau of Economic Research, March 2007); John T. Hsu and others, "Unintended Consequences of Caps on Medicare Drug Benefits," *New England Journal of Medicine* 354 (June 2006): 2349–59; Stephen B. Soumerai and others, "Effects of Limiting Medicaid Drug-Reimbursement Benefits on the Use of Psychotropic Agents and Acute Mental Health Services by Patients with Schizophrenia," *New England Journal of Medicine* 331 (September 1994): 650–55; and Stephen B. Soumerai and others, "Effects of Medicaid Drug-Payment Limits on Admissions to Hospitals and Nursing Homes," *New England Journal of Medicine* 325 (October 1991): 1072–77.

20. Michael E. Chernew, Allison B. Rosen, and A. Mark Fendrick, "Value-Based Insurance Design," *Health Affairs* 26, Web Exclusive (March/April 2007): W196–203.

21. In its cost estimates of the Medicare Modernization Act of 2003 (H.R. 1, November 2003, available at www.cbo.gov/ftpdocs/48xx/doc4808/11-20-MedicareLetter.pdf), CBO estimated that the revenue associated with the income-related premium would be $1.8 billion in fiscal 2010. Less than six months after these estimates were published, the Medicare

trustees reported in the 2004 *Trustees Report* that revenue from Part B premiums for fiscal 2010 would be $68 billion.

22. Karen Davis and others, "Medicare Extra: A Comprehensive Benefit Option for Medicare Beneficiaries," *Health Affairs,* Web Exclusive (October 4, 2005): W442–54.

23. Bobby Jindal, "Medicare Supplemental Insurance," Testimony before the House Subcommittee on Health, Committee on Ways and Means, 107 Cong. 2 sess. (GPO, March 14, 2002) (http://waysandmeans.house.gov/Legacy/health/107cong/3-14-02/3-14jind.htm).

24. Despite efforts to avoid adverse selection, it is possible for average costs to be somewhat higher than if everyone enrolled and thus to imply some additional federal costs. It is also possible for average costs to be reduced because those who are particularly risk averse would tend to enroll disproportionately, and there is some evidence that the risk-averse have lower-than-average health care costs. See Amy Finkelstein and Kathleen McGarry, "Multiple Dimensions of Private Information: Evidence from the Long-Term Care Insurance Market," *American Economic Review* 96 (September 2006): 938–58.

25. Eliot Fisher and others, "The Implications of Regional Variation in Medicare Spending. Part 1: The Content, Quality, and Accessibility of Health Care," *Annals of Internal Medicine* 138 (February 2003): 273–87.

26. Institute of Medicine, Committee on Redesigning Health Insurance Performance Measures, Payment, and Performance Improvement Programs, *Rewarding Provider Performance: Aligning Incentives in Medicare* (Washington: National Academies Press, 2007); Eliot Fisher and Karen Davis, "Pay for Performance—Recommendations of the Institute of Medicine," *New England Journal of Medicine* 355 (September 2006): e14 (http://content.nejm.org/cgi/content/full/NEJMp068216/DC1); and Donald M. Berwick, Nancy Ann Min DeParle, and David M. Eddy, "Paying for Performance: Medicare Should Lead," *Health Affairs* 22 (November/December 2003): 8–10.

27. Stephen Campbell and others, "Quality of Primary Care in England with the Introduction of Pay for Performance," *New England Journal of Medicine* 357 (July 2007): 181–90; Tim Doran and others, "Pay-for-Performance Programs in Family Practice in the United Kingdom," *New England Journal of Medicine* 355 (July 2006): 375–84.

28. Stuart Gutterman and Michelle P. Serber, *Enhancing Value in Medicare: Demonstrations and Other Initiatives to Improve the Program* (New York: Commonwealth Fund, January 2007).

29. Numerous papers have been written on options for Medicare drug design. See, for example, Richard G. Frank and Joseph P. Newhouse, *Mending the Medicare Prescription Drug Benefit: Improving Consumer Choices and Restructuring Purchasing* (Brookings Hamilton Project, April 2007).

30. Ibid.

31. Christopher Lee, "Experts Fault House Bill on Medicare Drug Prices," *Washington Post,* January 11, 2007, p. A14.

32. Patricia M. Danzon and Jonathan D. Ketcham, "Reference Pricing of Pharmaceuticals for Medicare: Evidence from Germany, the Netherlands, and New Zealand," in *Frontiers in Health Policy Research,* vol. 7, edited by Alan M. Garber and David M. Cutler (Cambridge, Mass.: MIT Press, 2003); and Panos Kanavos and Uwe Reinhardt, "Reference Pricing for Drugs: Is It Compatible with U.S. Health Care?" *Health Affairs* 22 (May/June 2003): 16–30.

33. Robert M. Wachter, "Expected and Unanticipated Consequences of the Quality and Information Technology Revolutions," *Journal of the American Medical Association* 295 (June 2006): 2780–83.

34. Thomas Lee and James Mongan, "Are Healthcare's Problems Incurable? One Integrated Delivery System's Program for Transforming Its Care," Health Policy Issues and Options Series, 2006-02 (Brookings, 2006); Adam Oliver, "The Veterans Health Administration: An American Success Story?" *Milbank Quarterly* 85 (November 2007): 5–35; and CBO, *The Health Care System for Veterans: An Interim Report* (December 2007).

35. See, for example, Northern New England Cardiovascular Disease Study Group (www.nnecdsg.org).

36. For an example of regional forums designed to harness local market forces in quality-of-care improvement, see the Regional Market Project within the Robert Wood Johnson Foundation's Aligning Forces for Quality program (www.forces4quality.org).

37. Karen Davis, "Learning from High Performance Health Systems around the Globe," testimony in *Health Care Coverage and Access: Challenges and Opportunities*, Hearing before the Senate Health, Education, Labor, and Pensions Committee, 110 Cong. 1 sess. (GPO, January 10, 2007) (www.commonwealthfund.org/usr_doc/996_Davis_learning_from_high_perform_hlt_sys_around_globe_Senate_HELP_testimony_01-10-2007.pdf); Christof Veit, "National Hospital Quality Benchmarking in Germany," Summary for the Commonwealth Fund, October 2005 (www.commonwealthfund.org/usr_doc/Veit_summary.pdf).

38. As health care spending grows continually, the savings although large, would come to only about 2 percent of health care spending. See Richard Hillestad and others, "Can Electronic Medical Record Systems Transform Health Care? Potential Health Benefits, Savings, and Costs," *Health Affairs* 24 (September/October 2005): 1103–17.

39. Roger Taylor and others, "Promoting Health Information Technology: Is There a Case for More Aggressive Government Action?" *Health Affairs* 24 (September/October 2005): 1234–45.

40. Stuart Butler and others, "Crisis Facing HCFA and Millions of Americans," *Health Affairs* 18 (January/February 1999): 8–10.

41. For a description of payment issues for Medicare Advantage plans, see Mark Merlis, "Medicare Payments and Beneficiary Costs for Prescription Drug Coverage," Medicare Policy Project Issue Brief (Menlo Park, Calif.: Kaiser Family Foundation, March 2007) (www.kff.org/medicare/upload/7620.pdf).

42. America's Health Insurance Plans, *Low-Income and Minority Beneficiaries in Medicare Advantage Plans, 2004* (Washington: Center for Policy and Research, February 2007).

43. Berenson, "Doctoring Health Care II."

44. Calculated from CMS, "2008 Enrollment Information," February 2008 (www.cms.hhs.gov/PrescriptionDrugCovGenIn).

45. Robert Pear, "Medicare, in a Different Tack, Moves to Link Doctors' Payments to Performance," *New York Times,* December 12, 2006, p. 27.

46. Elizabeth A. McGlynn and others, "The Quality of Health Care Delivered to Adults in the United States," *New England Journal of Medicine* 348 (June 2003): 2635–45.

47. Bruce C. Vladeck, "Plenty of Nothing—A Report from the Medicare Commission," *New England Journal of Medicine* 340 (May 1999): 1503–06.

## Chapter 5

1. The term "premium support" was coined by Henry J. Aaron and Robert D. Reischauer, in "The Medicare Reform Debate: What Is the Next Step?" *Health Affairs* 14 (Winter 1995): 8–30. It was adopted and modified by the National Bipartisan Commission on the Future of Medicare, *Building a Better Medicare for Today and Tomorrow* (March 16, 1999) (http://medicare.commission.gov/medicare/bbmtt31599.html). Other names for similar approaches include "competitive defined benefit," the term the Clinton administration used to describe its 1999 proposal, and "comparative cost adjustment," the language used to describe the premium support demonstration mandated by the 2003 Medicare Modernization Act. See National Economic Council, "President Clinton's Plan to Modernize and Strengthen Medicare for the 21st Century" (http://clinton2.nara.gov/WH/New/html/medicare.pdf). See also Jeff Lemieux, "The Breaux-Frist Legislative Proposal," Editorial (Washington: Progressive Policy Institute, November 1, 1999) (www.ppionline.org/ppi_ci.cfm?contentid=706&knlgAreaID=111&subsecid=141); Stuart M. Butler, Robert E. Moffit, and Brian M. Riedl, "Cost Control in the Medicare Drug Bill Needs Premium Support, Not Trigger," Backgrounder 1704 (Washington: Heritage Foundation, November 10, 2003) (www.heritage.org/Research/HealthCare/BG1704.cfm).

2. Alain C. Enthoven, *Health Plan: The Only Practical Solution to the Soaring Cost of Medical Care* (Reading, Mass.: Addison Wesley, 1980). See also Alain C. Enthoven and Richard Kronick, "Universal Health Insurance through Incentives Reform," *Journal of the American Medical Association* 265 (May 1991): 2532–36.

3. Aaron and Reischauer, "The Medicare Reform Debate."

4. In addition to risk adjustment, the MMA authorized "risk corridors" to protect plans and the government against large mis-estimates of cost and "reinsurance" for high-cost enrollees.

5. For a discussion of this form of competitive pricing, see Bob Berenson, "From Politics to Policy: A New Payment Approach in Medicare Advantage," *Health Affairs*, Web Exclusive (March 4, 2008):W156–64.

6. This requirement resembles that governing the State Children's Health Insurance Program.

7. The potential implications of these different choices are significant. In 2007, for example, average annual projected Medicare spending per beneficiary ranged from $9,600 in Louisiana to $6,360 in New Mexico, with the variation even wider at the county level. Congressional Budget Office (CBO), "Medicare Advantage Statistics by State," Letter to Senator Ron Wyden (April 17, 2007); CBO, *Designing a Premium Support System for Medicare* (December 2006).

8. If the Medicare subsidy were tied to per capita income, the proportion of health care spending covered by Medicare would fall by 21 percent after a decade and 40 percent after two decades. This statement presumes that per beneficiary expenditures under premium support grow about as fast as general health expenditures, as expenditures under traditional fee-for-service Medicare have done.

9. By contrast, the least costly half of beneficiaries accounted for only 3 percent of fee-for-service spending. MedPAC, *A Data Book: Healthcare Spending and the Medicare Program* (June 2007), p. 10.

10. Risk adjustment algorithms are subject to continuous study and improvement.

11. For a review of risk selection and risk adjustment, see Wyand P. M. M. Van de Ven and Randall P. Ellis, "Risk Adjustment in Competitive Health Plans," in *Handbook of Health Economics*, vol. 1A, edited by Anthony Culyer and Joseph Newhouse (Amsterdam: Elsevier, 2000), pp. 755–846. See also Joseph P. Newhouse, "Reimbursing Health Plans and Health Providers: Efficiency in Production versus Selection," *Journal of Economic Literature* 34 (September 1996): 1236–63.

12. Marian V. Wrobel and others, "Predictability of Prescription Drug Expenditures for Medicare Beneficiaries," *Health Care Financing Review* 25 (Winter 2003): 37–46.

13. For example, information is collected on such items as the fraction of each plan's participants receiving breast cancer screening and beta-blockers after heart attacks and practitioner turnover. These instruments are refined periodically. They will be used in the future to examine how various plans manage care for patients with chronic conditions, whether staffing in various specialties is adequate, and how the health care outcomes in various plans compare. The Centers for Medicare and Medicaid Services (CMS) disseminates summary quality information about certain plans in each area to help beneficiaries make informed choices (www.medicare.gov/MPPF/Include/DataSection/Questions/ListPlanByState.asp). The Health Care Effectiveness and Data Information Set (HEDIS), a tool used to measure performance, consists of seventy-one measures across eight domains of care. More than 90 percent of health plans use HEDIS, and many report results to payers and consumers.

14. The text example refers to a particular variant of premium support. We indicate where alternative arrangements have been considered.

15. Robert H. Miller and Harold S. Luft, "HMO Plan Performance Update: An Analysis of the Literature, 1997–2001," *Health Affairs* 21 (July/August 2002): 63–86.

16. See Daniel L. McFadden, "Free Markets and Fettered Consumers," *American Economic Review* 96 (March 2006): 5–29; Colin F. Camerer, "Prospect Theory in the Wild," in *Choices, Values and Frames*, edited by Daniel Kahneman and Amos Tversky (Cambridge University Press, 2000), pp. 288–300; Richard H. Thaler, "Mental Accounting Matters," *Journal of Behavioral Decision Making* 12 (September 1999): 183–206; and Jeffrey Liebman and Richard Zeckhauser, "Simple Humans, Complex Insurance, Subtle Subsidies," paper presented at an Urban/Brookings Tax Policy Center conference (Washington, February 2008) (www.taxpolicycenter.org/tpccontent/healthconference_zeckhauser.pdf).

17. As of March 2008, sufficient data to compare clinical measures in Medicare Advantage with similar measures in the traditional fee-for-service program did not exist. However, valid comparisons from a 2004 survey did show that fee-for-service beneficiaries were more likely than Medicare Advantage enrollees to give higher ratings for the quality of their health care and satisfaction with their health plan. MedPAC, *Medicare Payment Policy* (2008), pp. 259–60.

18. The challenge of multiple payers with different quality standards is explored in Sally Trude, Melanie Au, and Jon B. Christianson, "Health Plan Pay-for-Performance Strategies," *American Journal of Managed Care* 12 (September 2006): 537–42. Few studies have examined the relationship between competition and quality, but several have looked at the literature comparing quality in managed care plans and in unmanaged or loosely managed plans. See, for example, Miller and Luft, "HMO Plan Performance Update."

19. One indication of this is the cross-state correlations between dimensions of quality in fee-for-service Medicare and Medicare Advantage plans. Where Medicare Advantage quality tends to be high so does fee-for-service quality.

20. Jeanne M. Lambrew, "'Choice' in Health Care: What Do People Really Want?" Issue Brief (New York: Commonwealth Fund, September 2005).

21. In the early to mid-1990s, Medicare rates were about two-thirds of commercial payment rates for physician services, but since 1999 Medicare rates have consistently been in the neighborhood of 80 percent of commercial rates. Enrollment shifts in the private market from higher-paying indemnity plans to lower-paying health maintenance organizations accounted for much of the narrowing between Medicare and private insurance rates from the mid-1990s to 2001. Averaged across all services and areas, 2006 Medicare rates were 81.3 percent of extrapolated private rates compared with 82.6 percent in 2005. MedPAC, *Medicare Payment Policy* (2008), p. 89.

22. For a discussion of this potential effect, see CBO, *Designing a Premium Support System for Medicare.*

23. National Bipartisan Commission on the Future of Medicare, Memorandum from Senator John Breaux, "Subject: Premium Support Estimate from the HCFA Actuary," February 23, 1999 (http://thomas.loc.gov/medicare/premium.htm).

24. National Bipartisan Commission on the Future of Medicare, Memorandum from Jeff Lemieux, "Subject: Cost Estimate of the Breaux-Thomas Proposal," March 14, 1999 (http://thomas.loc.gov/medicare/cost31499.html).

25. CBO, *Designing a Premium Support System for Medicare.*

26. Jonathan Oberlander, "Is Premium Support the Right Medicine for Medicare?" *Health Affairs* 19 (September/October 2000): 84–99.

## Chapter 6

1. The term appears to have been first used by President George W. Bush in 2002. See White House, Office of the Press Secretary, "President Promotes Retirement Security Agenda," Remarks by the President at the 2002 National Summit on Retirement Savings, February 28, 2002 (www.whitehouse.gov/news/releases/2002/02/20020228-3.html). For a description of policies, see White House, Office of the Press Secretary, "Fact Sheet: America's Ownership Society: Expanding Opportunities," August 9, 2004 (www.whitehouse.gov/news/releases/2004/08/20040809-9.html). Also David Boaz, "Defining an Ownership Society" (Washington: Cato Institute, February 2005) (www.cato.org/special/ownership_society/boaz.html).

2. Consumers would "reap the full benefits and bear the full costs of decisions they make." Peter J. Ferrara, "Medical Savings Accounts: A Solution to Finance Health Care?" *USA Today Magazine* (May 1996); John C. Goodman, "Health Savings Accounts," Testimony before the Senate Finance Committee, Subcommittee on Health, 109 Cong. 2 sess., September 26, 2006, p. 7.

3. Centers for Medicare and Medicaid Services (CMS), Office of Public Affairs, "CMS Announces Steps to Improve Access to Consumer-Directed Health Plans in Medicare," Press Release, July 10, 2005 (www.cms.hhs.gov/apps/media/press/release.asp?Counter=1894).

4. Robert Nozick, *Anarchy, State, and Utopia* (New York: Basic Books, 1974).

5. Kenneth E. Thorpe and David H. Howard, "The Rise in Spending among Medicare Beneficiaries: The Role of Chronic Disease Prevalence and Changes in Treatment Intensity," *Health Affairs* 25 (September/October 2006): W378–88.

6. Michael Cannon, "Combining Tax Reform with Health Care Reform in Large HSAs," Cato Institute, *Tax and Budget Bulletin* 23 (May 2005) (www.cato.org/pubs/tbb/tbb-0505-23.pdf).

7. Jane Zhang, "Growing Pains of Private Medicare Plans," *Wall Street Journal,* May 8, 2007, p. A6.

8. American Medical Association, Council on Medical Service, "Critical Expansion of Medical Savings Accounts," Report 10, I-99 (Chicago, 1999).

9. For example, MSAs were a centerpiece of the alternative to the Clinton plan proposed by House Republican Minority Leader Robert Michel: the Affordable Health Care Now Act of 1994 (H.R. 3080).

10. Budget Reconciliation Bill, H.R. 2491, 104 Cong. 1 sess., 1995.

11. Alexandra Minicozzi, "Medical Savings Accounts: What Story Do the Data Tell?" *Health Affairs* 25 (January/February 2006): 256–67.

12. The idea was also applied to Medicaid in subsequent legislation. The Deficit Reduction Act of 2005 created a "Health Opportunity Account" demonstration program, under which up to ten states could create accounts linked to high deductibles (up to $2,500 for adults) for Medicaid services. The account would not need to pay for the deductible in full. If deemed successful after five years, the secretary of health and human services was authorized to extend the program nationwide.

13. These rules are more favorable than those that apply to Individual Retirement Accounts, 401k plans, or qualified pensions. They raise serious issues for tax policy, as account holders could use the proceeds of loans to deposit in health savings accounts. In practice, such interest is deductible, generating tax savings to the account holder. Since nothing about the health savings account itself is taxable, the net effect of the whole transaction—the loan plus the health savings account—is to reduce revenues. Thus health savings accounts are actively subsidized.

14. According to the 2007 EBRI/Commonwealth Fund Consumerism in Health Care Survey, 7.5 million adults ages 21–64 with private health insurance were enrolled in either a CDHP (a plan with an HSA or HRA) or an HDHP that was eligible to contribute to an HSA (up from 3.6 million in 2006). This represents 6.6 percent of adults ages 21–64 with private insurance (up from 3.2 percent in 2006). The survey did not include children. This enrollment number is comparable to estimates published by other sources. Paul Fronstin and Sara R. Collins, "Findings from the 2007 EBRI/Commonwealth Fund Consumerism in Health Survey," Issue Brief #315 (Washington: Employee Benefit Research Institute, March 2008) (www.commonwealthfund.org/usr_doc/Fronstin_consumerism_survey_2007_issue_brief_FINAL.pdf). Another 2007 survey found that 10 percent of employers offered consumer-directed health plans, and 5 percent of workers took such options (1.9 million in HSA-qualified plans, and 1.9 million in related health reimbursement accounts). This total does not count the policies purchased in the nongroup, individual market. Kaiser Family Foundation/Health Research and Educational Trust, *Employer Health Benefits 2007* (Menlo Park, Calif., 2007).

15. Government Accountability Office (GAO), *Federal Employees Health Benefits Program: First-Year Experience with High-Deductible Health Plans and Health Savings Accounts,* GAO-06-271 (GPO, 2006).

16. Some cost sharing could result from balance billing. MSA plans, like the traditional Medicare program, would require providers who choose to treat a Medicare beneficiary to accept as payment in full the applicable Medicare payment amount. Exceptions apply, however. Nonparticipating providers or providers who do not accept assignment on a particular claim are permitted to "balance-bill" the beneficiary, up to Medicare's applicable balance billing limits. These are generally limited to 15 percent of the applicable Medicare payment amount. Notably, nearly all physicians participating in Medicare are enrolled in the Medicare "participating physicians" program under which they sign an agreement that precludes them from balance-billing their Medicare patients, while hospitals and other institutional provider types are precluded by law from balance-billing Medicare beneficiaries. For a detailed description of MSAs, see Beth Fuchs and Lisa Potetz, "Medicare Consumer-Directed Health Plans," Medicare Issue Brief (Menlo Park, Calif.: Kaiser Family Foundation, March 2007).

17. This flexibility included the ability to offer coverage of preventative services during the deductible period, a deductible below the out-of-pocket maximum, cost sharing up to the out-of-pocket maximum, and cost differentials between in- and out-of-network services. Fuchs and Potetz, "Medicare Consumer-Directed Health Plans."

18. In 2008, plans were available in all fifty states and the District of Columbia, as well as Puerto Rico, Guam, and the U.S. Virgin Islands. CMS, *Part D Enrollment Data* (Washington, March 2008).

19. One bill would allow people in HSAs who turn sixty-five to opt out of Medicare and stay in their plans, with Medicare contributing its subsidy to the account. See *Health Care Choices for Seniors Act,* S. 2601, 109 Cong. 2 sess., 2006.

20. CMS, Office of Public Affairs, "Medicare Advantage Medical Savings Account (MSA) Plan Demonstration Proposal," Press Release, July 10, 2006 (www.cms.hhs.gov/apps/media/press/release.asp?Counter=1894).

21. The Medicare demonstration required that it be at least $2,000 per enrollee in 2008. This amount was below the maximum deductible of $10,500. CMS, "Your Guide to Medicare Medical Savings Account Plans" (Baltimore, February 2008) (www.medicare.gov/Publications/Pubs/pdf/11206.pdf). Note that most private insurance includes separate deductibles for individuals and for families or couples. Medicare has traditionally been strictly individual insurance. We retain that convention here.

22. CMS, "MSA Plans by State 2008" (www.cms.hhs.gov/MSA/Downloads/MSAhandbookMSA_changes120407r3.pdf).

23. CMS, "Your Guide to Medicare Medical Savings Account Plans" (Baltimore, February 2008) (www.medicare.gov/Publications/Pubs/pdf/11206.pdf).

24. Expenses that qualify for tax-free withdrawals from HSAs are listed in Internal Revenue Service, "Publication 502: Medical and Dental Expenses" (2007) (www.irs.gov/publications/p502/index.html).

25. CMS, "Helping Patients Get the Best Care for their Needs," Fact Sheet, June 1, 2006 (www.cms.hhs.gov/apps/media/press/release.asp?Counter=1872).

26. This sum is equal to the minimum deductible used in the Medicare demonstration. Congressional Budget Office (CBO), *High-Cost Medicare Beneficiaries* (Washington, May

2005). Inflation-adjusted from 2005 to 2008 dollars using the consumer price index for medical care services. See Bureau of Labor Statistics, Consumer Price Index–All Urban Consumers (Current Series) (www.bls.gov/CPI).

27. For a description of the Medicare Advantage system, see chapter 2. Note that in the current demonstration neither the requirements to return 25 percent of savings to beneficiaries nor the geographic adjustment of payments based on enrollees' residences applies.

28. In 2008, the amount deposited into beneficiaries' standard MSAs ranged from $1,250 to $1,725 per person. CMS, "MSA Plans by State 2008" (www.cms.hhs.gov/MSA/Downloads/MSAhandbookMSA_changes120407r3.pdf).

29. The nature of Medicare services and enrollees suggests that an index based on health spending for nonelderly people with different health needs may also have limitations. See CBO, *Technological Change and the Growth of Health Care Spending* (January 2008).

30. Calculations based on data from CMS, "National Health Expenditure Data: NHE summary including share of GDP, CY 1960–2006" (www.cms.hhs.gov/National HealthExpendData/02_NationalHealthAccountsHistorical.asp); and CBO, "Update of CBO's Economic Forecast," Letter to the Honorable Kent Conrad (February 15, 2008).

31. Paul Fronstin and Sara R. Collins, "Findings from the 2007 EBRI/Commonwealth Fund Consumerism in Health Survey," Issue Brief 315 (Washington: Employee Benefit Research Institute, March 2008) (www.commonwealthfund.org/usr_doc/Fronstin_con-sumerism_survey_2007_issue_brief_FINAL.pdf).

32. Board of Trustees, *2008 Annual Report of the Board of Trustees of the Federal Hospital Insurance and Federal Supplementary Medical Insurance Trust Funds* (Washington, 2008), table II.B1; MedPAC, *A Data Book: Healthcare Spending and the Medicare Program* (Washington, June 2007), p. 23; and Kaiser Family Foundation, "Medicare at a Glance," Fact Sheet (Menlo Park, Calif., February 2007) (www.kff.org/medicare/upload/1066-10.pdf).

33. Medicaid consumer direction of personal assistance services (CD-PAS) is a growing trend. Although overall enrollment in these programs is small, forty-two states offered consumer direction in Medicaid in 2006. These programs allow Medicaid beneficiaries control over hiring, scheduling, training, and paying of personal care attendants. For a review of CD-PAS efforts in California, Colorado, New York, and Virginia, see Henry Claypool and Molly O'Malley, *Consumer Direction of Personal Assistance Services in Medicaid: A Review of Four State Programs* (Washington: Kaiser Commission on Medicaid and the Uninsured, March 2008). This policy could be structured along the lines of the care coordination models being considered for chronically ill beneficiaries. MedPAC, *Report to the Congress: Promoting Greater Efficiency in Medicare* (Washington, June 2007). A different model has been tested in Medicaid demonstrations such as the "cash and counseling" demonstration and the Independence Plus waivers. See Barbara Phillips and others, *Lessons from the Implementation of Cash and Counseling in Arkansas, Florida, and New Jersey: Final Report* (Washington: Mathematica Policy Research, June 2003); Jeffrey S. Crowley, *An Overview of the Independence Plus Initiative to Promote Consumer-Direction of Services in Medicaid* (Washington: Kaiser Commission on Medicaid and the Uninsured, November 2003).

34. "Special needs plans" (SNPs) were created under the Medicare Modernization Act to offer private plan options to medically vulnerable populations, including those dually eligible for Medicare and Medicaid, those who are institutionalized, and those with severe or disabling chronic conditions. For a two-year review of SNPs in Medicare, see James Verdier

and others, *Do We Know if Medicare Advantage Special Needs Plans Are Special?*
(Washington: Kaiser Commission on Medicaid and the Uninsured, January 2008).

35. The deductible experiences a corresponding rise to $2,200.

36. This price and others are taken from the online pharmacy, drugstore.com.

37. John T. Hsu and others, "Unintended Consequences of Caps on Medicare Drug
Benefits," *New England Journal of Medicine* 354 (June 2006): 2349–59.

38. Stephen B. Soumerai and others, "Effects of Limiting Medicaid Drug-
Reimbursement Benefits on the Use of Psychotropic Agents and Acute Mental Health
Services by Patients with Schizophrenia," *New England Journal of Medicine* 331 (September
1994): 650–55; and Stephen B. Soumerai and others, "Effects of Medicaid Drug-Payment
Limits on Admissions to Hospitals and Nursing Homes," *New England Journal of Medicine*
325 (October 1991): 1072–77.

39. Allison B. Rosen and others, "Cost-Effectiveness of Full Medicare Coverage of
Angiotensin-Converting Enzyme Inhibitors for Beneficiaries with Diabetes," *Annals of
Internal Medicine* 143 (July 2005): 89–99.

40. This example is reported by Joseph P. Newhouse in "Reconsidering the Moral
Hazard-Risk Aversion Tradeoff," presidential address to the American Society of Health
Economists (http://healtheconomics.us/conference/2006/plenaries/powerpoint/newhouse-
madison.ppt).

41. John Gist, *A Profile of Older Taxpayers* (Washington: American Association of
Retired Persons, Public Policy Institute, September 2002) (http://assets.aarp.org/rgcen-
ter/econ/dd76_taxpayers.pdf).

42. The legislation governing health savings accounts permits deposits of up to $2,900
for individuals and $5,800 for families, as long as they are enrolled in a plan with a
deductible of at least $1,100 for individuals and $2,200 for families.

43. See, for example, *Universal Health Care Choices and Access Act,* S. 1019, 110 Cong.
1 sess., 2007.

44. For a detailed examination of these issues in the context of Social Security, see
National Academy of Social Insurance, *Uncharted Waters: Paying Benefits from Individual
Accounts in Federal Retirement Policy,* Study Panel Final Report (Washington, January 2005)
(www.nasi.org/usr_doc/Uncharted_Waters_Report.pdf).

45. Greg Scandlen and Phillips L. Gausewitz, "Bringing Health Savings Accounts to
Medicare" (Alexandria, Va.: Consumers for Choices in Health Care, September 2005)
(www.chcchoices.org/publications/HSAs%20in%20Medicare.pdf).

46. Michael F. Cannon, "Fix Medicare—Not Its Prices," *New York Post,* October 10,
2006.

47. Joseph P. Newhouse and the Insurance Experiment Group, *Free for All? Lessons from
the RAND Health Insurance Experiment* (Harvard University Press, 1993); J. P. Newhouse,
"Consumer-Directed Health Plans and the RAND Health Insurance Experiment," *Health
Affairs* 23 (November/December 2004): 107–13. See also Robyn Tamblyn and others,
"Adverse Events Associated with Prescription Drug Cost-Sharing among Poor and Elderly
Persons," *Journal of the American Medical Association* 285 (January 2001): 421–29; Tom
Rice and K. Y. Matsuoka, "The Impact of Cost-Sharing on Appropriate Utilization and
Health Status: A Review of the Literature on Seniors," *Medical Care Research and Review* 16
(December 2004): 415–52.

48. Amitabh Chandra, Jonathan Gruber, and Robin McKnight, "Patient Cost-Sharing, Hospitalization Offsets, and the Design of Optimal Health Insurance for the Elderly," Working Paper 12972 (Cambridge, Mass.: National Bureau of Economic Research, March 2007). The authors analyze the impact of cost sharing on the elderly in a modern setting, using a recent policy change in the California Public Employees Retirement System (CalPERS), a program that provides insurance to 1.2 million workers, retirees, and their dependents. The policy change consisted of staggered co-payment increases that affected different patient populations, those enrolled in an HMO and those in a PPO, at different times. The authors examine the effect of this change on use, comparing patients who were or were not exposed to the increase. A $10 increase in the office visit was associated with almost a 20 percent reduction in visits. A $7 to $8 increase in the average drug co-payment reduced drug use by 20 percent for HMO patients and by 6 percent for PPO patients (for HMO patients the increased co-payment applied to both generic and branded drugs; for PPO patients it applied only to branded drugs). The implied elasticities are substantially larger than those reported in the RAND HIE for the nonelderly, often exceeding 1 in absolute value.

49. This difference was statistically significant at $p \leq 0.05$ or better. Paul Fronstin and Sara R. Collins, "Findings from the 2007 EBRI/Commonwealth Fund Consumerism in Health Survey," Issue Brief 315 (Washington: Employee Benefit Research Institute, March 2008) (www.commonwealthfund.org/usr_doc/Fronstin_consumerism_survey_2007_issue_brief_FINAL.pdf).

50. Ibid.

51. According to the same survey, 22 percent of adults with deductibles of $1,000 or more took on credit card debt to pay for medical bills. Sara R. Collins, Jennifer L. Kriss, and others, *Squeezed: Why Rising Exposure to Health Care Costs Threatens the Health and Financial Well-Being of American Families* (New York: Commonwealth Fund, September 2006).

52. Regina E. Herzlinger, "Consumer-Driven Health Care: Freeing Providers to Innovate," *Healthcare Financial Management* 58 (March 2004): 66–68.

53. Evidence suggests that publicly releasing performance data stimulates quality improvement activity at the hospital level. Constance H. Fung and others, "Systematic Review: The Evidence That Publishing Patient Care Performance Data Improves Quality of Care," *Annals of Internal Medicine* 148 (January 2008): 111–23.

54. Atul A. Gawande, Robert J. Blendon, Mollyann Brodie, and others, "Does Dissatisfaction with Health Plans Stem from Having No Choices?" *Health Affairs* 17 (September/October 1998): 184–94; Karen Davis and others, "Choice Matters: Enrollees' Views of Their Health Plans," *Health Affairs* 14 (Summer 1995): 99–112.

55. This dissatisfaction did not translate to perceived quality of care or choice of doctors. For this measure, rates of satisfaction were comparable among enrollees in consumer-directed and comprehensive plans. Fronstin and Collins, "Findings from the 2007 EBRI/Commonwealth Fund Consumerism in Health Survey."

56. Quality information available to enrollees was limited. GAO, *Federal Employees Health Benefits Program: First-Year Experience with High-Deductible Health Plans and Health Savings Accounts,* GAO-06-271 (GPO, 2006), p. 26.

57. Fronstin and Collins, "Findings from the 2007 EBRI/Commonwealth Fund Consumerism in Health Survey." Yet focus groups conducted by the GAO found that few

HSA participants researched the cost of services before obtaining care. Some who asked doctors about costs found that the doctors themselves did not know.

58. The study results suggest that increases in hospital spending offset 20 percent of the savings from higher co-payments on physicians and prescription drugs. Amitabh Chandra, Jonathan Gruber, and Robin McKnight, "Patient Cost-Sharing, Hospitalization Offsets, and the Design of Optimal Health Insurance for the Elderly." See also Stephen T. Parente, Roger Feldman, and Jon B. Christianson, "Evaluation of the Effect of a Consumer-Driven Health Plan on Medical Care Expenditures and Utilization," *Health Services Research* 39 (August 2004): 1189–209.

59. America's Health Insurance Plans, *A Survey of Preventive Benefits in Health Savings Account Plans* (Washington: Center for Policy and Research, July 2007) (www.ahipresearch.org/pdfs/HSA_Preventive_Survey_Final.pdf).

60. Michael E. Chernew, Allison B. Rosen, and Mark Fendrick, "Rising Out-of-Pocket Costs in Disease Management Programs," *American Journal of Managed Care* 12 (March 2006): 150–54.

61. One analysis found that more than 95 percent of spending by privately insured households is attributable to people whose spending exceeds the minimum HSA deductible. Linda Blumberg and Leonard Burman, "Most Households' Medical Expenses Exceed HSA Deductibles," *Tax Notes,* August 16, 2004.

62. CBO, *High-Cost Medicare Beneficiaries* (May 2005). For historical data on the medical services component of the consumer price index, see Bureau of Labor Statistics, Consumer Price Index—All Urban Consumers (Current Series) (www.bls.gov/CPI).

63. G. C. Halvorsen, "Commentary—Current MSA Theory: Well-Meaning but Futile," *Health Services Research* 39(4), Part II (August 2004): 1119–22 (www.academy-health.org/publications/hsr.pdf). Average as well as marginal cost sharing may fall under consumer-directed health insurance, if it includes an effective stop-loss provision. See Dahlia K. Remler and Sherry A. Glied, "How Much More Cost Sharing Will Health Savings Accounts Bring?" *Health Affairs* 25 (July/August 2006): 1070–078.

64. CMS, National Health Expenditure Data (www.cms.hhs.gov/National HealthExpendData); Mark E. Litow, "Medicare versus Private Health Insurance: The Cost of Administration" (Milliman Inc., January, 6, 2006) (www.cahi.org/cahi_contents/resources/pdf/CAHIMedicareTechnicalPaper.pdf).

65. Ibid.

66. Aamer Baig, Jeff Nuckols, and Amy Dawson, *Insight: Seizing the HSA Opportunity: Developing a Winning Strategy to Grow Profits and Market Share in a Time of Transition* (Chicago: DiamondCluster, 2005).

67. Abundant evidence indicates that sick patients have both a deep yearning to trust their doctors and an aversion to relying on contrary information from other sources. Ha Tu and J. Lee Hargraves, "Seeking Health Care Information: Most Consumers Still on the Sidelines," Issue Brief 61 (Washington: Center for Studying Health System Change, 2003); Mark A. Hall, "Law, Medicine, and Trust," *Stanford Law Review* 55 (November 2002): 463–528; M. Gregg Bloche, "Trust and Betrayal in the Medical Marketplace," *Stanford Law Review* 55 (November 2002): 919–54.

68. Bloche believes that even with increased demand, there is more reason for doubt than optimism about the quality of discernible comparative performance information. He writes that "the complexity and individualized nature of clinical decision making have long

frustrated efforts to reduce medical judgment to algorithms, usable by either lay people or physicians to outperform doctors' case-by-case assessments. . . . The absence of science-based answers to most of the questions doctors face in daily practice . . . renders impossible the crafting of a comprehensive set of clinical decision rules (and quality benchmarks)." Bloche, "Trust and Betrayal in the Medical Marketplace," p. 1320.

## Chapter 7

1. Commonwealth Fund, *The Commonwealth Fund Health Care Opinion Leaders Survey: Assessing Health Care Experts' Views on Medicare and Its Future* (New York, July 2005).

2. Karen Davis and others, "Medicare versus Private Insurance: Rhetoric and Reality," *Health Affairs*, Web Exclusive (October 9, 2002): W311–24.

3. For an explanation of integrated delivery's contribution to high-quality care and of the increase in the gap between the care that medical science can deliver and what it is now delivering in the United States, see Thomas Lee and James Mongan, "Are Healthcare's Problems Incurable? One Integrated Delivery System's Program for Transforming Its Care," Health Policy Issues & Options Series, 2006-02 (Brookings, 2006); and Thomas Lee, James Mongan, and Robert Mechanic, "Transforming U.S. Health Care: Policy Challenges Affecting the Integration and Improvement of Care," Health Policy Issues & Options Series, 2006-01 (Brookings, 2006).

4. Amy Finkelstein, "The Aggregate Effects of Health Insurance: Evidence from the Introduction of Medicare," *Quarterly Journal of Economics* 112 (February 2007): 1–37.

5. Lengths of stay have fallen in many other countries as well, but those in the United States are among the lowest in the world. See Gerald F. Anderson, Bianca K. Frogner, and Uwe E. Reinhardt, "Health Spending in OECD Countries," *Health Affairs* 26 (September/October 2007): 1481–89.

6. Joseph P. Newhouse, "Reimbursing Health Plans and Health Providers: Selection versus Efficiency in Production," *Journal of Economic Literature* 34 (September 1996): 1236–63.

7. Thomas Lee, James Mongan, and Robert Mechanic, "Transforming U.S. Health Care: Policy Challenges Affecting the Integration and Improvement of Care," Health Policy Issues & Options Series, 2006-01 (Brookings, 2006); and Elliott S. Fisher and others, "Creating Accountable Care Organizations: The Extended Hospital Medical Staff," *Health Affairs* 26, Web Exclusive (December 5, 2006): W44–57.

8. See, for example, Constance H. Fung and others, "Systematic Review: The Evidence That Publishing Patient Care Performance Data Improves Quality of Care," *Annals of Internal Medicine* 148 (January 2008): 111–23; Judith H. Hibbard, Jean Stockard, and Martin Tusler, "Does Publicizing Hospital Performance Stimulate Quality Improvement Efforts?" *Health Affairs* 22 (March/April 2003): 84–94; Rachel M. Werner and David A. Asch, "The Unintended Consequences of Publicly Reporting Quality Information," *Journal of the American Medical Association* 293 (March 2005): 1239–44.

9. Research has not found that the quality of care in managed care plans is demonstrably better than that in different financing and delivery systems. Robert H. Miller and Harold S. Luft, "HMO Plan Performance Update: An Analysis of the Literature, 1997–2001," *Health Affairs* 21 (July/August 2002): 63–86.

10. Paul Fronstin and Sara R. Collins, "Findings from the 2007 EBRI/Commonwealth Fund Consumerism in Health Survey," Issue Brief 315 (Washington: Employee Benefit Research Institute, March 2008) (www.commonwealthfund.org/usr_doc/Fronstin_consumerism_survey_2007_issue_brief_FINAL.pdf).

11. Ibid.

12. MedPAC, *Report to the Congress: Medicare Payment Policy* (Washington, March 2008), p. 54; and Government Accountability Office, *Medicare Physician Fees: Geographic Adjustment Indices Are Valid in Design, but Data and Methods Need Refinement* (March 2005), p. 4.

13. Joseph P. Newhouse, *Pricing the Priceless: A Healthcare Conundrum* (MIT Press, 2002).

14. To the extent that plans collude over bids, the benchmark (or weighted average of plan bids) that serves as the basis of the government payment might be higher than it could be with a strict defined benefit.

15. See Joseph P. Newhouse and the Insurance Experiment Group, *Free for All? Lessons from the RAND Health Insurance Experiment* (Harvard University Press, 1993); J. P. Newhouse, "Consumer-Directed Health Plans and the RAND Health Insurance Experiment," *Health Affairs* 23 (November/December 2004): 107–13; and Amitabh Chandra, Jonathan Gruber, and Robin McKnight, "Patient Cost-Sharing, Hospitalization Offsets, and the Design of Optimal Health Insurance for the Elderly," Working Paper 12972 (Cambridge, Mass.: National Bureau of Economic Research, March 2007).

16. Jonathan Oberlander, *The Political Life of Medicare* (University of Chicago Press, 2003).

17. Allowing Medicare to negotiate drug prices became part of the "100-hour" legislative package passed by the newly Democratic House of Representatives in January 2007. The drug industry and administration countered with a major public relations campaign whose basic message was, "The market is working." Americans in general and seniors in particular support the idea that Medicare should negotiate for drug prices; in November 2006, 67 percent of seniors strongly favored the idea, with another 14 percent somewhat favoring it (www.kff.org/kaiserpolls/upload/7604.pdf).

18. Editorial Board, "Medagogues," *Washington Post*, September 15, 1995, p. A24.

19. Theda Skocpol, *Boomerang: Clinton's Health Security Effort and the Turn against Government.* (New York: W. W. Norton, 1996).

20. White House, Office of the Press Secretary, "President's Remarks to the Coalition for Medicare Choices," May 17, 2002 (www.whitehouse.gov/news/releases/2002/05/20020517-8.html).

21. Jill Bernstein and Rosemary A. Stevens, "Public Opinion, Knowledge, and Medicare Reform," *Health Affairs* 18 (January/February 1999): 180–93.

22. Fronstin and Collins, "Findings from the 2007 EBRI/Commonwealth Fund Consumerism in Health Survey."

23. Steve Machlin and Marc Zodet, "Out-of-Pocket Health Care Expenses by Age and Insurance Coverage, United States, 2003," Statistical Brief 126 (Rockville, Md.: Agency for Healthcare Research and Quality, May 2006) (www.meps.ahcpr.gov/mepsweb/data_files/publications/st126/stat126.pdf)

24. Congressional Budget Office (CBO), *The Budget and Economic Outlook: Fiscal Years 2008 to 2018* (January 2008); and Organization for Economic Cooperation and Development, *OECD Health Data 2007* (Paris, October 2007).

25. Richard Foster, "The Financial Outlook for Medicare," Testimony before the House Subcommittee on Health, Committee on Ways and Means, 110 Cong. 2 sess. (GPO, April 1, 2008) (http://waysandmeans.house.gov/media/pdf/110/RSFTestimony.pdf).

26. Board of Trustees, *2008 Annual Report of the Board of Trustees of the Federal Hospital Insurance and Federal Supplementary Medical Insurance Trust Funds* (Washington, 2008), table III.A3.

27. CMS, National Health Expenditure Projections (www.cms.hhs.gov/NationalHealth ExpendData).

# Appendix A

1. In 2006 there were 392 LTCHs (359 urban) with 130,164 cases and a payment per case of $34,859. Medicare spending on LTCHs was $4.5 billion in that year (about 1 percent of total), a 66 percent increase from the first full year of the PPS in 2003. Medicare beneficiaries accounted for about 70 percent of these hospitals' revenues in 2006. LTCHs are not distributed evenly throughout the nation. The five states with the largest number of LTCH beds per thousand Medicare beneficiaries account for 40 percent of the available beds but only 12 percent of the Medicare beneficiary population. Relatively new LTCHs—those that entered the Medicare program under the PPS—have frequently located in markets where LTCHs already existed instead of opening in new markets. The evidence on quality is mixed. Risk-adjusted rates of death in LTCHs and readmission to acute-care hospitals fell from 2004 to 2006, as have risk-adjusted rates of death within thirty days of discharge, albeit at a slower rate. Over the same period, patients experienced fewer instances of postoperative sepsis, pulmonary embolisms, or deep vein thromboses but more decubitus ulcers and infections due to medical care. MedPAC, *Report to the Congress: Medicare Payment Policy* (March 2008), pp. 217–28.

2. In 2006 there were 1,224 LTCHs (969 urban) with 404,255 cases and a payment per case of $15,354. Medicare spending on LTCHs was $6 billion in that year (about 1.5 percent of total), only a 6 percent increase since 2002 when the PPS was implemented for these services. Medicare beneficiaries accounted for about 70 percent of IRF cases in 2006. IRFs use the "functional independence measure" to gauge the physical and cognitive functioning of the patient, as well as the burden imposed on caregivers. Although the case mix of IRF patients increased considerably between 2004 and 2007, all patients increased their functioning from admission to discharge, from 22.8 in 2004 to 23.8 in 2007. The subset of Medicare patients who were discharged home increased functioning between admission and discharge from 25.0 in 2004 to 27.5 in 2007. In 2007 the most frequent diagnoses for beneficiaries in IRFs was stroke, representing about 21 percent of all cases. Relatively few Medicare beneficiaries use these services (less than 1 percent) because they must generally be able to tolerate and benefit from three hours of therapy per day to be eligible for treatment. MedPAC, *Report to the Congress: Medicare Payment Policy* (2008), pp. 195–204.

3. In 2006 there were 2,200 IPFs with 499,000 cases and a payment per case of about $8,000. Medicare spending on IPFs was $4 billion in that year (about 1 percent of total),

with Medicare beneficiaries accounting for about 30 percent of psychiatric facilities' revenue. MedPAC, *Medicare Payment Basics: Psychiatric Hospital Services Payment System* (October 2007).

4. MedPAC, *A Data Book: Healthcare Spending and the Medicare Program* (June 2007), p. 124.

5. Before 2002, LTCHs and IRFs were paid under the Tax Equity and Fiscal Responsibility Act of 1982, on the basis of their average costs per discharge, up to an annually adjusted facility-specific limit. Under the PPS, discharges are assigned to case-mix groups containing patients with similar clinical problems that are expected to require similar amounts of resources. Each case-mix group has a national relative weight reflecting the expected costliness of treatment for a patient in that category compared with that for the average LTCH or IRF patient. The PPS payment rates cover all operating and capital costs that LTCHs and IRFs would be expected to incur in furnishing covered services. The initial payment level (base rate) for a typical discharge in the 2008 rate year is $38,356 for LTCHs and $13,451 for IRFs. The base rate is adjusted for market area wages by multiplying the labor-related portion of the base payment amount—76 percent—by a version of the hospital wage index and the result is added to the nonlabor portion. The sum is then case-mix-adjusted by multiplying the local base rate by the relative weight for the case-mix group to create the PPS payment rate for each patient. Both payment systems have an outlier policy for patients with short stays and for high-cost patients whose costs exceed a fixed-loss threshold. MedPAC, *Medicare Payment Basics: Long-Term Care Hospitals Payment System* (October 2007); and MedPAC, *Medicare Payment Basics: Rehabilitation Facilities (Inpatient) Payment System* (October 2007).

6. Before 2005, Medicare also paid IPFs under the Tax Equity and Fiscal Responsibility Act of 1982 on the basis of their average costs per discharge, as long as they did not exceed the facility-specific limit that was adjusted annually. The base payment rate for each patient day in an IPF is based on the national average daily routine operating, ancillary, and capital costs in IPFs in 2002. For the 2008 rate year, the base payment rate is $615 per day. MedPAC, *Medicare Payment Basics: Psychiatric Hospital Services.*

# Appendix B

1. Cancer, children's, and sole community hospitals receive special hold-harmless payments if their revenues from the outpatient prospective payment system are less than they would have been under the pre-2000 payment system. MedPAC, *Medicare Payment Basics: Outpatient Hospital Services Payment System* (October 2007).

2. Services remain in these APCs for two to three years, while the Centers for Medicare and Medicaid Services (CMS) collects the data necessary to develop payment rates for them. Each year the CMS determines which new services, if any, should be placed in new-technology APCs. Payments for new-technology APCs are not subject to budget neutrality adjustments, so they increase total OPPS spending. MedPAC, *Medicare Payment Basics: Outpatient Hospital Services.*

3. In 2008, Medicare began a four-year transition to a new payment system for ASCs based on the outpatient prospective payment system (OPPS). The ASC conversion factor will be based on a percentage of the OPPS conversion factor.

4. Aggregate outlier payments represented 42 percent of the Medicare outpatient revenues for the top 1 percent of hospitals with the most outlier claims in 2002. Three-quarters of outlier claims are for procedures receiving payments of $300 or less. See MedPAC, *Medicare Payment Policy: Report to the Congress* (March 2004), pp. 85–97. As of 2007, Medicare limits aggregate outlier payments to 1 percent of total OPPS payments. Outlier payments are made budget neutral by reducing the conversion factor by 1 percent. MedPAC, *Medicare Payment Basics: Outpatient Hospital Services*.

5. Total pass-through payments cannot be more than 2 percent of total OPPS payments in 2004 and beyond. Before the start of each calendar year, Medicare estimates total pass-through spending. If this estimate exceeds 2 percent of estimated total OPPS payments, the agency must reduce all pass-through payments in that year by a uniform percentage to meet the 2 percent threshold. Also, Medicare adjusts the conversion factor to make pass-through payments budget neutral. MedPAC, *Medicare Payment Basics: Outpatient Hospital Services*.

6. CMS, *Second Annual Report to Congress: Evaluation of Medicare's Competitive Bidding Demonstration for Durable Medical Equipment, Prosthetics, Orthotics, and Supplies* (September 2002); Government Accountability Office, *Past Experience Can Guide Future Competitive Bidding for Medical Equipment and Supplies* (GPO, September 2004); MedPAC, *Medicare Payment Basics: Durable Medical Equipment Payment System* (October 2007).

7. The system will start with ten metropolitan statistical areas (MSAs) in 2008 and expand to eighty MSAs by 2009.

8. The base rate is adjusted for age (younger than eighteen, eighteen to forty-four, forty-five to fifty-nine, sixty to sixty-nine, seventy to seventy-nine, and eighty or older) and two body measurement variables (body surface area and body mass index). MedPAC, *Medicare Payment Basics: Outpatient Dialysis Services Payment System* (October 2007).

9. The MMA and subsequent CMS regulations changed the way Medicare pays for dialysis drugs. As intended by policy, the payment rate for most dialysis drugs decreased while the prospective payment that CMS pays for each dialysis treatment increased. From 1996 to 2004, the use of dialysis drugs increased 15 percent annually, but decreased by 5 percent between 2004 and 2006. MedPAC, *Report to the Congress: Medicare Payment Policy* (March 2008), p. 120.

10. Ibid., pp. 124–25.

# Appendix C

1. For example, the conversion factor update for 2002 was 4.8 percent while the MEI was 2.6 percent. In 1998 the respective figures were 2.3 percent and 2.2 percent.

# Appendix D

1. The International Classification of Diseases, Ninth Revision, Clinical Modification (ICD-9-CM) is based on the World Health Organization's Ninth Revision, International Classification of Diseases (ICD-9). ICD-9-CM is the official system of assigning codes to diagnoses and procedures associated with hospital utilization in the United States. CMS,

ICD-9 Provider and   Diagnostic Codes, is available at www.cms.hhs.gov/ICD9
ProviderDiagnosticCodes.

2. MedPAC, *Report to the Congress: Medicare Payment Policy* (March 2000), pp. 71–74.

3. There are actually 746 categories; 2 are not used for payment. The new system has
335 base DRGs that reflect similar principal diagnoses and procedures. Most base DRGs are
further subdivided according to whether patients have no complication or co-morbidity
(CC), one or more CCs, or one or more major CCs. In the first year, payments will be based
on a 50/50 blend of MS-DRGs and the previous DRGs. MedPAC, *Medicare Payment
Basics: Hospital Acute Inpatient Services Payment System* (October 2007). Along with DRG
refinement, Medicare also implemented corresponding payment cuts over a five-year
period, including a 0.6 percent reduction for fiscal 2008, 0.9 percent for fiscal 2009, and
similar reductions through 2012. These reductions aim to offset the improved documenta-
tion and coding, and therefore payment, that Medicare believes providers will adopt according to past data. Chief actuary Richard Foster notes: "Substantial evidence supports our
conclusion that, absent such an adjustment, aggregate payments for inpatient hospital services would increase significantly under the new system—without any corresponding
growth in actual patient severity. If we didn't make this adjustment, the Medicare Part A
trust fund would be exhausted an estimated 18 months earlier than previously forecast."
CMS, "Final Changes to the Hospital Outpatient Prospective Payment System and CY
2008 Payment Rates," *Federal Register* 72 (227) (November 27, 2007): 66579–67226.
CMS, Office of Public Affairs, "CMS Announces Payment Reforms for Inpatient Hospital
Services in 2008" (August 1, 2007).

4. CMS, "Final Changes to the Hospital Inpatient Prospective Payment Systems and
Fiscal Year 2008 Rates," *Federal Register* 72 (162) (August 22, 2007): 47129–48175.

5. To qualify for outlier payments, a case must have costs greater than Medicare's payment rate for the case plus a "fixed loss" or cost threshold. Law requires that the secretary
of the Department of Health and Human Services set the cost threshold so that outlier payments for any year are projected to be not less than 5 percent or more than 6 percent of total
operating DRG payments plus outlier payments. Historically, the secretary has set the cost
threshold so that 5.1 percent of estimated inpatient PPS payments are paid as outliers.
When the number of DRGs is increased to 744 in fiscal 2008, many cases that were high-
cost outlier cases in 2007 could be paid as nonoutlier cases in 2008. For this reason, CMS
reduced the cost threshold from $24,485 in 2007 to $22,185 in 2008. Medicare pays 80
percent of the excess costs. CMS, "Final Changes to the Hospital Inpatient Prospective
Payment Systems and Fiscal Year 2008 Rates," *Federal Register* 72 (162) (August 22, 2007):
47129–48175; and CMS, "Revised FY08 IPPS Rates" (October 18, 2007). CMS also
makes outlier payment for costly individual services furnished by outpatient hospitals under
the outpatient PPS. In 2008 CMS defines an outlier as a service with costs that exceed 1.75
times the payment rate and that exceed the payment rate by $1,575. For a service meeting
both thresholds, CMS will reimburse the hospital for 50 percent of the difference between
the cost of furnishing the service and 1.75 times the payment rate. CMS also limits aggregate outlier payments to 1 percent of total OPPS payments. CMS, "Final Changes to the
Hospital Outpatient Prospective Payment System and CY 2008 Payment Rates," *Federal
Register* 72 (227) (November 27, 2007): 66579–67226.

6. The Medicare Modernization Act of 2003 (P.L. 108-173) required this moratorium.
The fiscal 2008 inpatient PPS rule requires physician-owned hospitals to disclose ownership

to patients and provide the names of the physician owners upon request. The rule also requires physician-owned hospitals to require physician owners who are members of the hospital's medical staff to disclose their ownership to the patients they refer to the hospital. Disclosure would be required at the time of referral. CMS, "Final Changes to the Hospital Inpatient Prospective Payment Systems and Fiscal Year 2008 Rates," 47129–48175.

7. Under Section 651 of H.R. 3162 (The Children's Health and Medicare Protection Act of 2007), Congress would impose a permanent ban on physician referrals of Medicare patients to new specialty hospitals in which they have an ownership interest, require existing hospitals to limit physician ownership to 40 percent, and limit individual physician ownership to 2 percent. It would also prohibit the addition of new inpatient beds and operating rooms in existing specialty hospitals that get Medicare reimbursement.

8. MedPAC, *Medicare Payment Basics: Hospital Acute Inpatient Services.*

9. A biological is any substance, such as a serum or vaccine, derived from animal products or other biological sources and used to treat or prevent disease.

# Index

Access and coverage: age of eligibility and, 46; coordination of, 116; decisions and determination of, 36, 167n28, 167n29; ensuring access, 31–33; expansion of covered services, 10, 12; general description of, 29, 51, 116; high-deductible plans and, 109–10; limits and reductions of, 36, 47, 116; Medicare Modernization Act and, 10; problems with, 170n49; public views of, 47. *See also* Reforms

Administration and management, 64–65. *See also* Reforms

Agency for Healthcare Research and Quality (U.S.), 56, 100

AMA. *See* American Medical Association

Ambulatory payment classification (APC) groups, 138–39, 188n2, 188n3

American Medical Association (AMA), 4, 18

APCs. *See* Ambulatory payment classification groups

Australia, 56

Balanced Budget Act of *1997* (BBA), 6–7, 17, 26

Baucus, Max (D-Mont.), 7

BBA. *See* Balanced Budget Act of *1997*

Benchmarks, 75, 77–78, 85, 89, 95–96, 99

Beneficiaries: age of, 171n56; approval of Medicare, 116; costs borne by, 2, 10, 78; eligibility of, 13–14; forgoing of care, 109–10; Medicare spending per beneficiary, 14; numbers of, 13. *See also* Reforms

Benefits: core benefits, 76; defined benefits, 53, 76, 117; extension of, 12–13; gaps in, 29, 31; limits on, 2; premium support and, 76–77; retiree health benefits, 10; Social Security Disability Insurance and, 12; taxes and, 43–44; uniformity of benefit structure, 51. *See also* Reforms

Bipartisan Commission on the Future of Medicare (*1999*), 68

Breaux, John (D-La.), 7

195

disproportionate share payments,153n22; DRGs and, 152n19; to health plans, 79; hold harmless payments, 188n1; for medical education, 16, 153n21; outlier payments, 16, 153n20, 189n4, 190n5; overpayments, 2, 26, 27, 67, 144, 163n82; pass-through payments, 16, 189n5; pay-for-performance (P4P) approach, 35; payment differentials, 63; per-capita spending, 5, 14, 38, 98, 99, 112; per-discharge payments, 16; per-procedure/input payments, 35, 59; pricing for outpatient services, 138–39; prospective payment system, 15–16, 17–18, 36, 117, 137, 138, 143–44, 154n25; risk-adjusting plan payments, 26; systems for special hospitals, 137; usual and customary fee schedules, 18. *See also* Financing and funding; Premiums

PBMs. *See* Pharmaceutical benefit managers

PDPs. *See* Prescription drug plans

Penalties, 49, 63, 64, 81, 95, 98, 125

PFFSs. *See* Private fee for service plans

Pharmaceutical benefit managers (PBMs), 60–61

Physical therapy, 66

Physicians: acceptance of Medicare patients, 32–33, 157n45, 165n10; charges/prices and billing of, 33, 40, 180n16; cost sharing and, 31–32; decisionmaking by, 80; growth in services of, 169n42; Medicare payments to, 18–19, 38, 41–42, 43, 157n47, 168n37, 170n48, 178n21; opposition to Medicare, 1, 18; patient satisfaction with, 168n33; physician-owned hospitals, 144, 190n6. *See also* Providers; Reforms

Political issues: categories of Medicare services, 14–15; costs of Medicare, 85; individual choice in health care, 94; Medicare Catastrophic Coverage Act, 5–6; Medicare, 4, 51, 53, 68; Medicare Modernization Act, 7–8; Part D prescription drug benefit, 7, 21; reforms, 56, 68, 114, 131–35, 137. *See also* Congress

Preferred provider organizations (PPOs), 27, 162n81, 163n82

Premiums: amounts of, 13; growth in, 47; Medicaid assistance with, 25; Medicare Catastrophic Coverage Act, 6; Medigap premiums, 161n69; premium support systems, 41, 49; prescription drug plans, 20

Premium support. *See* Reforms—premium support model

Prescription Benefits (Medicare). *See* Part D

Prescription drug plans (PDPs), 20, 159n58

Prescription drugs: adverse effects of, 166n17; free drugs, 56; history of coverage for, 2, 75; MMA and, 20; price negotiations for, 9, 61; reference pricing for, 61; tiered pricing, 61. *See also* Part D; Reforms

Preventive Services Task Force (U.S.), 55

Prices. *See* Costs; Financing and funding; Payments

Private insurance. *See* Insurance

Private fee for service plans (PFFSs), 162n77, 163n82

Private sector, 10, 22

Problems and shortcomings: cost control, 38–43; in coverage, 51; in financial access, 31–32; general description of, 2; quality and satisfaction, 33–37, 42–43, 51; reforms and, 32, 33, 37–38, 43–50, 51; structural shortcomings, 30–31; variation in service use, 42. *See also* Goals, performance and options

Providers: Balanced Budget Act and, 6; consumer-directed health care and, 94, 110; inaccurate billing and fraud by, 41; limiting prices of, 40–41; Medicare Modernization Act and, 8; Medicare rules and, 34–35, 62, 81; payments for services, 157n51, 190n3; programs opposed by, 2; programs supported by, 1; prospective payments to, 12–13, 36; selection and payment of, 81. *See also* Hospitals and hospital care; Physicians; Reforms

Public goods, 64

Public sector, 18. *See also* Parts A, B, C, D